walking *the* cape *and* islands

A COMPREHENSIVE GUIDE TO THE WALKING AND HIKING TRAILS OF CAPE COD, MARTHA'S VINEYARD, AND NANTUCKET

Walking

the Cape and

Islands

a comprehensive guide to
the walking and hiking trails
of Cape Cod, Martha's Vineyard,
and Nantucket

David Weintraub

MENASHA RIDGE PRESS
Birmingham, Alabama

Library of Congress Cataloging-in-Publication Data

Weintraub, David, 1949–
    Walking the cape and islands: a comprehensive guide to the walking and hiking
trails of Cape Cod, Martha's Vineyard, and Nantucket/David Weintraub.—1st ed.
        p. cm.
    ISBN 10: 0-89732-603-2
    ISBN 13: 978-0-89732-603-2
    1. Hiking—Massachusetts—Cape Cod—Guidebooks. 2. Hiking—Massachusetts—
Martha's Vineyard—Guidebooks. 3. Hiking—Massachusetts—Nantucket Island—
Guidebooks. 4. Walking—Massachusetts—Cape Cod. 4. Walking—Massachusetts—
Martha's Vineyard. 5. Walking—Massachusetts—Nantucket Island. 7. Cape Cod
(Mass.)—Guidebooks. 8. Martha's Vineyard (Mass.)—Guidebooks. 8. Nantucket
Island (Mass.)—Guidebooks. I. Title.

GV199.42.M42W45 2006
917.44'90444—dc22

                                                                    2006041857

Cover design by Travis Bryant
Text design by Annie Long and Karen Ocker
All photos © David Weintraub
Maps by Ben Pease

Menasha Ridge Press
P.O. Box 43673
Birmingham, AL 35243
www.menasharidge.com

TABLE OF CONTENTS

TABLE OF CONTENTS

TABLE OF CONTENTS

ACKNOWLEDGMENTS

Making a book is, for me, mostly a solo adventure, but many people lend support along the way. I am indebted to the following folks in various land-management agencies and organizations, both public and private, for their advice and expertise: Karen Beattie, Mike Brady, John Chatham, Matthew Dix, Gage Dobbins, Pat Dwyer, Kristen Fauteux, Sue Haley, Kim Heard, Jeanne Johnson, Keith Johnson, Richard W. Johnson, Chris Kennedy, James Lengyel, Alan S. Marcy, Jim Mitchell, Sue Moynihan, Dennis Murley, Diane Nickerson, Jon Peterson, Steve Prokop, Eric Savetsky, Julie Schaeffer, Bob Sherman, Martha Twombly, and John Varkonda.

I also offer a tip of my (ever present) hat to Ivan Ace, Mimi Ace, Tom Connell, Richard Johnson, Marsha Salett, and Nancy Wigley—Cape Cod friends whose love and knowledge of the natural world are always inspirational. This is my first book for Menasha Ridge Press, and I have enjoyed working with the crew there, especially Russell Helms, who provided a light but insightful editorial hand.

Finally, I want to thank my wife, Maggi Morehouse, whose love and support have encouraged me to wander the trails less traveled.

—*David Weintraub*

For Brewster and Mary Fox, and Bernie and Rory Greenhouse—
who welcome me home to Wellfleet each summer.

ABOUT THE AUTHOR

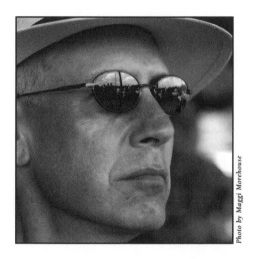

Photo by Maggi Morehouse

David Weintraub is a writer, photographer, and editor based in South Carolina and Cape Cod. His other books are *Adventure Kayaking: Cape Cod and Martha's Vineyard, Afoot & Afield: San Francisco Bay Area, Top Trails: San Francisco Bay Area, East Bay Trails, North Bay Trails, Monterey Bay Trails* (all published by Wilderness Press), and *Peninsula Tales and Trails* (Graphic Arts Books). David's articles and photographs have appeared in such magazines as the *American Bar Association Journal, Audubon, Backpacker, Entrepreneur, Forbes, Hemispheres, Photo District News, Sierra, Smithsonian,* and *Sunset,* and in books such as *San Francisco: The City's Sights and Secrets* (Chronicle Books), *The World of Shorebirds* (Sierra Club Books), and *Cape Cod on My Mind* (Falcon Publishing). David is an avid walker, birder, kayaker, and skier. Visit David on the Web at **www.weintraubphoto.com.**

PREFACE

This book is the result of field work that began in 2001 and continued through the summer of 2005. As with my *Adventure Kayaking: Cape Cod and Martha's Vineyard* (Wilderness Press), the impetus for writing this book was simple: no other comprehensive trail guide existed for Cape Cod, Martha's Vineyard, and Nantucket. Given the amount of beautiful open space, and a history of walking that dates back to Henry David Thoreau's visits, this was a void needing to be filled.

As a long-time summer resident of Wellfleet, a town on the Outer Cape, I already knew about nearby rambles in Cape Cod National Seashore and at Wellfleet Bay Wildlife Sanctuary. But for me, the woods of Falmouth, the hills of Martha's Vineyard, or the moors of Nantucket might as well have been on the moon. Just as working on the kayaking book exposed me to a watery wonderland, so walking the trails and byways of the Cape and Islands for this book showed me a wealth of open space to which I would—and in many cases did—eagerly return.

I learned to enjoy the outdoors on the West Coast, in Oregon and California. My first books were trail guides to the San Francisco Bay Area. When I began to walk the trails on the Cape and Islands for this book, I found I had to shift my mindset. For one thing, the beauty here is much more intimate, subtle, and less grounded on the grand vista: a reflection in a kettle pond takes the place of a Sierra summit. For another, in many cases the walking routes consist primarily of unsigned dirt roads and single-track trails which depart from unmarked trailheads beside obscure parking areas. Finally, although some agencies produce fine maps for their trails, this is by no means the rule. In fact, I considered (not entirely in jest) "I Got Lost So You Don't Have To" as the motto for this book.

Ah, but the rewards of walking the Cape and Islands are plentiful. There is great variety of terrain and scenery here—from the crashing Atlantic Ocean to pristine kettle ponds, from densely wooded tracts to open expanses of salt marsh, and from sandy shorelines to wildflower-carpeted grasslands. The diversity of habitats ensures a wide selection of vegetation and wildlife, and the Cape and Islands are great places to learn about plants and animals, especially birds. As an added treat, each season reveals a new face of the Cape and Islands; and the most-familiar one, the summer visage, is complemented by those of fall, winter, and spring.

So I hope you use this book in the spirit in which it was written—as a guide to the walking and hiking trails, but also as a guide to what makes the Cape Cod, Martha's Vineyard, and Nantucket such special places. I also hope that, once enamored of our precious open spaces, you will join in the effort to preserve, protect, and increase them.

INTRODUCTION

▶ CAPE COD AND THE ISLANDS

Where better to take a walk than on Cape Cod, Martha's Vineyard, or Nantucket, New England's seaside playground? Whatever your goal—fitness, family outing, nature study, or just a relaxing stroll—you'll find a walk to match it in the pages of this book. The walks described explore all of the Cape and Islands' habitats, including pine–oak forest, heathland, shrubland, grassland, freshwater wetland, salt marsh, and shoreline beach. They range in length from 0.4 miles to 11.2 miles, and in difficulty from easy to difficult.

Cape Cod National Seashore, part of the National Park Service, administers nearly 44,000 acres of public open space, the most on the Cape and Islands. Other agencies, including Massachusetts Department of Conservation and Recreation, Massachusetts Audubon Society, The Trustees of Reservations, Martha's Vineyard Land Bank Commission, Sheriff's Meadow Foundation, Nantucket Islands Land Bank, and Nantucket Conservation Foundation, have significant holdings. Finally, many of the Cape and Islands towns also own open space, as do town-associated conservation foundations.

Beyond walking and hiking, the best general-purpose guidebook for the Cape and islands is *Cape Cod, Martha's Vineyard, & Nantucket,* sixth edition (The Countryman Press) by Kim Grant. In it you will find information about lodging (including camping), dining, shopping, transportation, and sightseeing. Getting around the Cape and Islands by car can be challenging, especially during the busy summer months; having a good road atlas is essential. This book uses the street names in the excellent Official Arrow™ street atlas for Cape Cod, Martha's Vineyard, and Nantucket. *Note:* Public transportation serves many of the trailheads on Martha's Vineyard and Nantucket, but is not currently an option for trailheads on Cape Cod.

▶ GEOLOGY

Where tourists on the Cape and Islands today see idyllic beaches, gently rolling hills, and picturesque harbors, geologists see remnants of an icy past. Glacial activity was responsible for many of the area's most recognizable features, including Cape Cod's curved-arm configuration, Martha's Vineyard's and Nantucket's triangular shape, the Elizabeth Island chain bordering Buzzard's Bay, along with the popular wave-washed coastlines and plentiful freshwater ponds.

About 21,000 years ago, at the end of the Pleistocene Epoch, the Laurentide ice sheet, which covered part of North America, reached its maximum southward advance in the vicinity of present-day Nantucket and Martha's Vineyard. About 3,000 years later, as global temperatures rose, the glacier began to melt and retreat, raising sea levels and leaving behind various landforms, the most noticeable of which are end moraines, outwash plains, and kettles.

End moraines are ridges of soil and rocks pushed, lifted, and/or folded ahead of an ice sheet as it advances, and then left behind when it retreats. End moraines form the backbone of Cape Cod, Martha's Vineyard, and Nantucket. For example, the Buzzard's Bay moraine runs northeast through the Elizabeth Islands and along the east side of Buzzard's Bay. It joins the Sandwich moraine, which runs eastward from the Cape Cod Canal to

INTRODUCTION

roughly Yarmouth, or about halfway to the Atlantic shore. The uplands of Martha's Vineyard and Nantucket are also moraines.

The region's outwash plains formed when water from melting ice poured out of the ice sheet, carrying with it accumulated sand and gravel. As the name suggests, outwash plains are mostly flat, gently sloping landforms that decrease in elevation the farther one moves from the associated moraine. Most of the low-lying areas on the Cape and Islands consist of outwash plains.

Kettles formed when large blocks of ice broke off from the retreating ice sheet and were buried in an outwash plain. When the ice blocks eventually melted, they left depressions in the landscape. As the sea level rose the water table rose with it, flooding many of the kettles and forming kettle ponds. According to the USGS, there are about 353 lakes and ponds on Cape Cod, 62 on Martha's Vineyard, and 28 on Nantucket. These range in size from an acre or less to 1,157 acres (Edgartown Great Pond on Martha's Vineyard). Most kettle ponds are fairly shallow, but a few reach depths of more than 80 feet. A kettle pond open to salt water is called a salt pond.

Since the retreat of the Laurentide ice sheet, other forces, including wind, waves, and ocean currents, have been shaping the Cape and Islands, forming dunes, sea cliffs, beaches, barriers, and salt marshes.

For example, wind-transported sand particles deposited atop barrier spits formed the dunes of Sandy Neck (Barnstable) and the Province Lands (North Truro, Provincetown). The sea cliffs of Wellfleet and Truro, which rise to more than 150 feet above the Atlantic Ocean, as well as those on Martha's Vineyard and Nantucket, are the result of wave action eating into glacial deposits.

Waves, especially those associated with winter storms, and water currents can also create and reshape beaches, inlets, and offshore sandbars from year the year, removing sand from one area and depositing it elsewhere. When waves and water currents move sand lengthwise along a beach, this is called shore drifting. Elongated barriers—beaches, islands, and spits—are the result of shore drifting. Some examples include Nauset Beach and Provincetown's "hook" on Cape Cod; Cape Poge on Martha's Vineyard; and Great Point and Coatue on Nantucket.

Salt marshes form where a barrier protects a bay or tidal creek, allowing salt-tolerant plants to grow and trap sediments. This process eventually raises the elevation of the marsh, creating one of nature's richest ecosystems. Twice-daily high tides flood the marsh's lowest areas, but its highest zone is under water only during the highest tides of the month. The Great Marshes of Barnstable, protected by Sandy Neck, and Nauset Marsh in Eastham, protected by Coast Guard Beach, are two of the Cape's largest salt marshes.

(The material is this section is based on Robert N. Oldale's excellent book, *Cape Cod, Martha's Vineyard & Nantucket: The Geologic Story* (On Cape Publications).

▶ CLIMATE

The climate of the Cape and Islands is strongly influenced by the surrounding waters, primarily the North Atlantic Ocean. In summer, the ocean's relatively cool waters help moderate heat spreading north and east from the mainland. In winter the opposite it true: the ocean's waters provide a source of warmth relative to the cold air mass which settles over most of New England. Thus the Cape and Islands, on average, enjoy slightly milder temperatures, in both summer and winter, than the mainland.

For example, the average daily high temperature in July, the warmest month, for the Town of Barnstable on Cape Cod is 78° F. By comparison, the average daily high in July in Springfield, Massachusetts (also the warmest month there), which is in the Connecticut River Valley, is 85° F, or about 7° F warmer. But Barnstable's lowest average daily temperature, which occurs in January, is 21° F. This would seem almost balmy in Pittsfield, on the western edge of the state, which in January sees an average daily low of 13° F.

AVERAGE DAILY HIGH AND LOW BY MONTH FOR BARNSTABLE, MASS.
(Source: www.weather.com)

	JAN	FEB	MAR	APR	MAY	JUN
HIGH	37°	38°	44°	52°	62°	72°
LOW	21°	22°	29°	38°	48°	57°

	JUL	AUG	SEP	OCT	NOV	DEC
HIGH	78°	77°	71°	60°	51°	42°
LOW	63°	63°	55°	44°	37°	27°

Most visitors to the Cape and Islands come during July and August, but an increasing number of folks are discovering the pleasures of the "shoulder" months, including June, September, and October. And there are also those who relish the cold, crisp days of late autumn and winter.

July and August are the warmest months and also the most humid. Winds are generally from the southwest, increasing during the afternoons. Fog and haze may be present. After the passage of a cold front, cooler, clearer, and drier air infiltrates the region, but this respite usually lasts only a few days. The rumble of thunder is sometimes heard in the distance, but the frequent electrical storms that plague the mainland during the summer rarely make it east across Cape Cod Bay.

Many people consider September and October the Cape and Islands' best months for outdoor pursuits. Days are still relatively warm, but usually without summer's "hazy, hot, and humid" conditions. June can be highly variable—a mix of warm sunny days and cool, rainy ones. Spring often tries the patience of even the most die-hard native—who, having survived the winter, now yearns for a bit of warmth and sunshine and is instead rewarded more often than not with wind and rain.

The question of climate change is a tricky one, but in recent years the Cape and Islands have seen uncommonly cold, snowy winters and summers with long dry spells. In addition to blizzards, the weather hazards here include hurricanes and nor'easters. Besides damaging homes and toppling trees and powerlines, these potent storms also rearrange the landscape, especially along the coastline, where the wind, tide, and waves form a potent combination. (The last strong hurricane hit the Cape and Islands was Bob in 1991.)

Before setting off for a walk, it's a good idea to check the latest weather forecast and pay particular attention to any advisories, watches, and warnings. You can obtain frequently

INTRODUCTION

updated weather forecasts via the Internet—three sites used by the author are **www .my-cast.com, www.noaa.gov/wx.html,** and **www.weather.com.** You can also buy a special radio to receive NOAA weather broadcasts; these are available at Radio Shack and outdoor stores.

▶ PLANT COMMUNITIES

Unlike birds, plants have no standardized common names, which is why botanists and serious plant enthusiasts generally use scientific names, i.e. genus and species. For example, the same plant may have several common names, and the same common name may be used for more than one plant. In addition, some plants may have unique local names. So, the tree *Nyssa sylvatica*, which in this book is called tupelo, may also be dubbed sour gum, black gum, and, on Martha's Vineyard, beetlebung. The common names used in this book are distilled from several standard reference books, including *Newcomb's Wildflower Guide* (Little, Brown and Company) and *The Flora of Cape Cod* (The Cape Cod Museum of Natural History).

In *Common Trailside Plants of Cape Cod National Seashore,* Michael E. Whatley divides the Cape's plant communities, along with some of their typical plants, as follows (where different, plant names used in this book are in parentheses):

IMPOVERISHED SANDY SOIL, DUNES, HEATHLANDS American beach grass, dusty miller, broom crowberry, golden heather, poverty grass, seaside goldenrod, sweet fern, beach pea, lichen, and scrub oak.

UPLAND FORESTS, DRY AND OPEN WOODS Pitch pine, white oak, black oak black cherry, sassafras, black huckleberry, bearberry, checkerberry, star flower, and spotted wintergreen.

MOIST LOWLAND WOODS, DEVELOPED FORESTS American beech, tupelo, wild sarsaparilla, highbush blueberry, lowbush blueberry, sweet pepperbush, mayflower, winterberry, shadbush, southern arrowwood, inkberry, sheep laurel, and swamp azalea.

FRESHWATER PONDS, STREAMS Slender arrowhead, golden club, pickerelweed, white water lily, and meadowsweet.

FRESHWATER SWAMPS, RECEDING PONDS, SHALLOW BOGS Atlantic white cedar, red maple, buttonbush, American cranberry.

BACK DUNES, TRANSITIONAL FIELDS Beach plum, salt-spray rose, Virginia rose, common blackberry, poison ivy, bullbrier (greenbrier), and bayberry.

OPEN FIELDS, FOREST MARGINS Eastern red cedar, Virginia creeper, honeysuckle, wild asparagus, fox grape, and bouncing bet.

ALTERED, PREVIOUSLY CULTIVATED HABITATS Domestic apple, black locust, tree of heaven, and multiflora rose.

SALTWATER MARSHES Salt marsh (saltwater) cordgrass, salt meadow grass (salt hay), seaside lavender (sea lavender) glasswort, sea rocket, eelgrass, knotted wrack, and rockweed.

INTRODUCTION

▶ ANIMALS

The Cape and Islands are great places to observe and study wildlife. A variety of habitats attracts a wide range of species, ranging from the tiniest insects to mammals such as whitetail deer and coyotes, and seasonal changes contribute to the ever-changing array of fauna. The area is best known, however, for its birds, particularly migratory shorebirds, which pass through briefly in May on their way to breeding grounds in Canada and the Arctic, but then return in large numbers from about mid-July through September.

BIRDS

Many people consider birds to be the Cape and Islands' main wildlife attraction, and prime birding areas such as South Beach (Chatham), Nauset Marsh (Eastham), Wellfleet Bay Wildlife Sanctuary, and the Beech Forest (Provincetown), along with areas in Martha's Vineyard and Nantucket, attract visitors from across the United States and around the world. Although primarily known as a great area to see shorebirds in migration, the Cape and Islands also provide ideal habitat for seabirds, waterfowl, wading birds, birds of prey, and songbirds.

Seeing birds requires being in the right place at the right time: location, time of year, time of day, tides, and weather may all affect the outcome. If you are new to birding, the best way to learn is to go with an experienced birder or a birding group. Some of the agencies overseeing the open spaces described in this book—Cape Cod National Seashore and the Massachusetts Audubon Society, for example—sponsor birding walks and trips.

Several great resources exist for the do-it-yourself birder:

Birding Cape Cod (On Cape Publications). Published in 2005, this updated version of the classic guide contains town-by-town birding routes for the entire Cape, along with much other helpful information.

MassBird, www.massbird.org. A Web site dedicated to birding in Massachusetts, with bird sightings and links to bird books and journals, bird clubs, and weather and tide information.

The Birdwatchers General Store, (800) 562-1512, **www.birdwatchersgeneral store.com.** Located at 32 Route 6A in Orleans, just south of Stop and Shop, this venue provides one-stop shopping for all your birding needs, including optics, field guides, bird feeders, and bird-related gifts.

Cape Cod Bird Club, www.massbird.org/ccbc. Founded in 1972, this is one of the largest bird clubs in New England, with 500 members. The club meets at the Cape Cod Museum of Natural History in Brewster on the second Monday of each month, September to May, and also conducts walks on and off Cape.

Approximately 360 species of birds have been recorded on Martha's Vineyard, including more than 60 so-called accidentals (five or fewer sightings). The Nantucket list has about 350 species, including more than 50 accidentals. The latest *Checklist of the Birds of Cape Cod* (2002) shows 317 species of birds having been recorded at least ten times in the last 20 years. According to *Birding Cape Cod*, about 130 of these are local nesters. *Birding Cape Cod* sorts characteristic breeding bird species by habitat; the habitats and a few of the common species are as follows:

INTRODUCTION

RESIDENTIAL AREAS Mourning dove, Carolina wren, American robin, gray catbird, chipping sparrow, song sparrow, northern cardinal, eastern kingbird, northern mockingbird, brown-headed cowbird, Baltimore oriole, and house finch.

FIELDS, PASTURES, MOORS, AND EDGES Eastern kingbird, tree swallow, eastern bluebird, northern mockingbird, yellow warbler, prairie warbler, red-winged blackbird, and American goldfinch.

ALL WOODLANDS Red-tailed hawk, great horned owl, downy woodpecker, northern flicker, blue jay, common crow, and black-capped chickadee.

PITCH PINE BARRENS Hermit thrush, pine warbler, prairie warbler, eastern towhee, and chipping sparrow.

MIXED PINE-OAK WOODLANDS Eastern screech-owl, red-bellied woodpecker, eastern wood pewee, great crested flycatcher, tufted titmouse, white-breasted nuthatch, and Baltimore oriole.

FRESHWATER MARSHES Mute swan, Canada goose, American black duck, mallard, belted kingfisher, yellow warbler, common yellowthroat, swamp sparrow, and red-winged blackbird.

SALT MARSHES Osprey, American oystercatcher, willet, and saltmarsh sharp-tailed sparrow.

DUNES AND BEACHES Piping plover, herring gull, great black-backed gull, common tern, and least tern.

MAMMALS

Except for an occasional squirrel or rabbit, you probably won't see too many mammals while walking on the Cape and Islands, especially if you visit during the summer and explore the trails only during midday. Many of the area's mammals are nocturnal, most avoid being out during the heat of the day, and nearly all shun contact with humans.

Some of the common land mammals here include eastern chipmunks, coyotes, whitetail deer, red foxes, white-footed mice, muskrats, raccoons, eastern cottontails, striped skunks, squirrels (eastern gray, red), meadow voles, and woodchucks. Marine mammals include Atlantic white-sided dolphins, finback whales, humpback whales, minke whales (also called piked whales), northern right whales, pilot whales (also called blackfish), and seals (harbor, gray).

REPTILES AND AMPHIBIANS

The Cape and Islands have no poisonous snakes, but it is still unwise to handle any snake, as it may bite (this applies to all wildlife). Present here are the northern water snake, northern redbelly snake, eastern garter snake, eastern hognose snake, northern ringneck snake, northern black racer, and eastern milk snake.

Turtles include snapping turtle, spotted turtle, eastern box turtle, eastern painted turtle, common musk turtle, and northern diamondback terrapin. Sea turtles, including Kemp's ridley, loggerhead, and green, sometimes become "cold-stunned" and strand on the beaches of Cape Cod Bay, usually during November and December.

INTRODUCTION

Salamanders are represented here by three species: redback salamander, spotted salamander, and red-spotted newt. Frogs and toads include eastern spadefoot, American toad, Fowler's toad, northern spring peeper, gray treefrog, bullfrog, green frog, wood frog, and pickerel frog.

Note: Some of the reptiles and amphibians found on Cape Cod may be missing from Martha's Vineyard and/or Nantucket.

▶ HUMAN HISTORY

The modern tourist era, which began on the Cape and Islands after World War II, is just one facet of the area's fascinating history. When Thoreau made the three visits (1849, 1850, 1855) to Cape Cod that provided material for his book of the same name, he found "a wild, rank place" imbued with "naked Nature"; a place where, he wrote, "My spirits rose in proportion to the outward dreariness." Although hardly the text for a tourism brochure, Thoreau's book, now considered a classic of nature writing, inspired an interest in the "bared and bended arm of Massachusetts," where "A man may stand . . . and put all America behind him."

Tourism developed slowly on the Cape and Islands, taking root from early nineteenth-century Methodist camp meetings in Wellfleet, Eastham, Oak Bluffs, and elsewhere, and also from hunting and fishing camps that dotted the landscape from Sandwich to Monomoy. Getting to and around the Cape prior to 1848, when rail service from Boston to Sandwich was established, involved traveling by boat and/or stagecoach. By 1873, however, the Cape Cod Railroad was running trains all the way to Provincetown. Ferry service provided access from several Cape towns to Martha's Vineyard and Nantucket, which were reeling from the collapse of the whaling industry.

The railroad provided an important new source of revenue just when the region's economic foundation, based primarily on the sea, was declining. The 1870s saw the beginning of a tourism-based economy that continues to this day. Ironically, it was the area's seafaring past, complete with whaling ships, fishing boats, and "old salts," that provided nostalgic grist for books, magazine article, and even picture postcards touting the Cape and Islands' appeal as a seaside destination.

Soon wealthy Boston "Brahmins" were building summers homes in Upper Cape towns such as Falmouth, Bourne, and Cotuit, while hotels, inns, and cottages sprang up from Woods Hole to Provincetown. "Gentleman gunners" flocked to the bays and salt marshes to shoot waterfowl and shorebirds. Meanwhile, in Provincetown, a lively arts scene formed around the Cape Cod School of Art, founded in 1899, and the Provincetown Players, which opened 1916 with *Bound East for Cardiff,* a play by the as-yet-undiscovered Eugene O'Neill.

By the "roaring" 1920s, the automobile was doing what the railroad had done some 50 years earlier: changing the way people got to and around Cape Cod. Opened in 1935, the Bourne and Sagamore bridges across the Cape Cod Canal facilitated auto travel from the mainland. The Depression and World War II interrupted the steady rise of tourism, but not for long. After the war, the Cape began to modernize its roadways to accommodate the

INTRODUCTION

boom in visitors, who were enjoying newfound prosperity and vacation time. Other facilities, such as motels, resort communities, shops, and restaurants, quickly followed.

Today the Cape and Islands are dealing with the fallout from what was largely uncontrolled and unplanned growth: declining water quality, traffic congestion, soaring home prices, lack of affordable housing, loss of habitat for wildlife. Fortunately, various federal, state, and local agencies, along with nonprofit organizations, have made preserving the character of Cape Cod their top priority. For example, Cape Cod National Seashore, established in 1961, protects nearly 44,000 acres of open space on the Outer Cape. State and local agencies, along with private land trusts, have protected thousands of additional acres.

The land's original inhabitants, Native Americans, are known to have been in the area around 9,000 years ago. When explorers such as Bartholomew Gosnold, Samuel de Champlain, and others visited the region in the early 1600s, they encountered the Wampanoags, whose territory stretched from Narragansett Bay, in present-day Rhode Island, east to the Atlantic Ocean, and included Martha's Vineyard and Nantucket. The Wampanoags lived in villages; hunted, fished, and raised crops; and used fire to clear fields and keep tracts open for wildlife.

Although the name "Cape Cod" was bestowed by Gosnold, many other familiar local names—Mashpee, Nauset, Pamet, for example—are Wampanoag, which means "People of the East." When the Pilgrims aboard the *Mayflower* landed in Provincetown harbor on November 11, 1620, they encountered not an uninhabited wilderness but, in the words of Henry C. Kittredge, Cape Cod's great historian, "an organized community . . . inhabited by generation after generation of natives."

Under the leadership of Capt. Myles Standish, some of the Pilgrims made three exploratory trips, one by land and two by small boat, or shallop. During these trips the Pilgrims took some corn they found buried near present-day Corn Hill in Truro, helped themselves to some utensils from an abandoned Wampanoag home, and fired some shots at a group of Native Americans at First Encounter Beach in present-day Eastham. On the third trip, a fierce blizzard severely damaged the shallop, but luck was with the Pilgrims and they washed up in Plymouth. In effect, they put the Cape behind them.

By the late 1630s however, settlers began arriving on the Cape, coming first to Sandwich (incorporated in 1639), which had an extensive salt marsh that provided fodder for cattle, forests that furnished lumber, and a creek that supplied herring and water for a mill. Settlement began on Martha's Vineyard with the founding of what is now Edgartown in 1642, and on Nantucket in 1659. As settlement spread throughout the Cape and Islands, a subsistence economy—farming, grazing, hunting, and fishing—prevailed.

The sea had always been an important source of food for both the Native Americans and the Europeans. Cod, mackerel, and other fish lured Cape fishermen to Georges Bank off the coast of New England and then to the Grand Banks off Newfoundland and Labrador. Provincetown had a large fishing fleet, and other towns with good harbors had busy waterfronts and fleets of their own.

But it was the sperm whale, prized for its clean-burning oil and fragrant ambergris, which brought fame and wealth to the islands of Nantucket and Martha's Vineyard. From around 1715, when deep-sea whaling began to take the place of near-shore pursuits,

INTRODUCTION

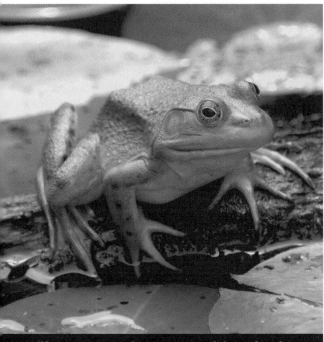

Bullfrogs are among the common amphibians found on the Cape and Islands.

through the era of around-the-world whale hunting on factory ships, chronicled by Herman Melville in *Moby-Dick,* the Islands reaped the benefits of the Leviathans' slaughter. A series of events, including Nantucket's Great Fire of 1846, the opening of commercial oil fields in Pennsylvania in 1859, and the Civil War, topped the Islands from the pinnacle of worldwide whaling.

The North Atlantic off of Cape Cod has been the graveyard for an estimated 3,000 vessels, many of which were wrecked on the area's treacherous shoals and storm-tossed beaches. Starting in 1746 with the establishment of Brant Point Light in Nantucket, about 40 lighthouses were erected on the Cape and Islands to warn mariners of the dangers that lay close to shore.

In 1872, Congress created the U.S. Life Saving Service, which eventually became the Coast Guard, and a dozen stations were built along the Atlantic shore from the southern tip of Monomoy, off Chatham, to Race Point in Provincetown. In 1914, an idea first conceived of by the early settlers was realized: the opening of the Cape Cod Canal, which links Cape Cod Bay and Buzzards Bay and provides a relatively safe sea route between Boston and New York.

▶ GETTING THERE AND AROUND

Cape Cod is located on the southeast coast of Massachusetts, roughly equidistant from Boston and Providence, RI. The Cape Cod canal, which is spanned by two highway bridges, divides the Cape from the mainland. Martha's Vineyard and Nantucket are islands south of Cape Cod. Thus, the Cape is accessible by road, by air, and by boat; the islands are accessible by air and by boat.

A complete listing of car-free ways to reach the Cape and Islands, and to get around once there, is provided by the Cape Cod Chamber of Commerce at **www.smartguide.org.**

INTRODUCTION

Links to airlines, bus lines, and boats serving the Cape and Islands are on the Smart Guide Web site. Web URLs and phone numbers of these carriers are also in Appendix C (page 280).

Road access to Cape Cod from Boston is via Interstate 93 and Route 3 to the Sagamore Bridge. From Providence, Rhode Island, take Interstate 195 and Route 25 to the Bourne Bridge. Once on the Cape, there are three major roadways: Route 6, which runs the length of the Cape from the Sagamore Bridge to Provincetown; Route 6A, running from Sagamore to Orleans, north of and generally parallel to Route 6, and then again from Truro to Provincetown, southwest and then south of Route 6; and Route 28, which runs from the Bourne Bridge to Falmouth, Hyannis, Chatham, and Orleans.

Boat access to Martha's Vineyard from Cape Cod is via Falmouth–Edgartown Ferry, Hy-Line Cruises, Island Queen, Patriot Party Boats, and The Steamship Authority (the only line that can accommodate cars and trucks). Air service to the Vineyard from Cape Cod and elsewhere is provided by Cape Air and US Airways Express. Web URLs and phone numbers for all of the above are in Appendix C.

The major roadways on Martha's Vineyard are as follows: in Aquinnah (Gay Head), State Road; in Chilmark, North, Middle, and South roads; in West Tisbury, North, Middle, State, Old County, and Edgartown–West Tisbury roads; in Tisbury, State and Edgartown–Vineyard Haven roads; in Oak Bluffs, Seaview Avenue and Edgartown–Vineyard Haven and Beach roads; and in Edgartown, Edgartown–West Tisbury, Edgartown–Vineyard Haven, East Vineyard Haven, and Beach roads.

Boat service to Nantucket from Cape Cod is via Freedom Cruise Lines, Hy-Line Cruises, and The Steamship Authority (the only line that can accommodate cars and trucks). Air service to the island from Cape Cod and elsewhere is provided by Cape Air, Continental Express, Island Airlines, Nantucket Airlines, and US Airways Express. Web URLs and phone numbers for all of the above are in Appendix C.

On Nantucket, the major roadways going westward from Nantucket Town are Cliff, Madaket, and Hummock Pond roads; going southward is Surfside Road; and going eastward are Milestone, Monomoy, and Polpis roads.

Note: Public transportation is available to some of the trailheads on Martha's Vineyard and Nantucket, but private cars are still the way most people on Cape Cod reach their destinations. Hopefully this will change in coming years with the expansion of bus and shuttle service and the introduction of new routes. The Cape has several wonderful bicycle trails, including one that runs from Harwich to Wellfleet, connecting Nickerson State Park and Cape Cod National Seashore. Bicycles are popular on Martha's Vineyard and Nantucket, and both islands have bicycle routes and paved bike trails.

▶ ENJOYING THE TRAILS

Enjoying the Cape and Islands on foot requires only a minimal amount of preparation, a bit of attention to comfort and safety, and an awareness of trail etiquette. A little care and consideration, along with the appropriate attire and footwear, will go a long way toward making your walk—and everyone else's—an enjoyable one. (For more on all these topics, see the following pages.)

INTRODUCTION

Most of the walks described in this book follow dirt roads, dirt walking paths, dirt single-track trails, paved paths, sandy beaches—or some combination of these. In places, wooden boardwalks aid in crossing swampy or wet areas, and sometimes wooden steps help you negotiate steep sections. So your feet, for the most part, will be following a prepared surface and not tromping across uncharted terrain.

Even though volunteers assist with maintaining many of the trails, not all the trails on the Cape and Islands are in perfect condition. The routes described herein all follow official trails—none involves bushwhacking—but that doesn't ensure the absence of poison ivy, greenbrier, downed limbs, and other hazards or obstructions. Most trailheads have no facilities (restrooms, water, etc.), and maps, if available, may be sketchy or obsolete. Many of the dirt roads and trails described in this book lack signage.

If you enjoy group walks, there are agencies and groups that organize and/or lead outings on the Cape and Islands. Among these are Appalachian Mountain Club, Cape Cod Bird Club, Cape Cod National Seashore, Cape Cod Pathways, Martha's Vineyard Land Bank Commission, and Wellfleet Bay Wildlife Sanctuary. See Appendix C for Web URLs and phone numbers.

BEFORE YOU GO

Preparing for a walk on the Cape and Islands is often as simple as choosing a route and journeying to the trailhead. During the summer months, lightweight clothing, supportive footwear (running shoes work fine), a hat for sun protection, water, and a snack may be all you need. Spring and fall walks may require the addition of a windbreaker or rain jacket, an insulating vest, sweater, or jacket, lightweight gloves, and a warm cap or headband. If you venture out during the coldest months, bundle up, wear warm socks and boots, and keep your neck and head warm (your mother was right, as always).

In recent years, mobile phone coverage has improved dramatically on the Cape and Islands, but there are still areas where phones don't work. Therefore, it is unwise to rely solely on a mobile phone in case of an emergency. If you feel concerned—for example, if you have a medical condition or are walking alone and not used to doing so—let someone know the location of the trailhead, the make/model of your car, the route you are planning to follow, and when you expect to return.

Note: Directions to the trailhead, along with other directions in the route description, are given by compass, so it is a good idea to carry one.

COMFORT AND SAFETY

The Cape and Islands are fairly benign places to venture out of doors—no grizzly bears, no poisonous snakes, no towering rock cliffs or crevassed glaciers to cross. A new generation of lightweight, breathable fabrics makes it possible to protect yourself against ticks and other biting insects, poison ivy, and sunburn while staying comfortable. In fact, the biggest threat to life and limb may be driving to the trailhead, especially during the busy summer months. The precautions recommended on the next several pages will help you avoid the relatively few hazards found here.

INTRODUCTION

TICKS

Ticks, and especially the tick that carries Lyme disease, present the most serious health hazard for walkers on the Cape and Islands. Fortunately, there are half a dozen simple steps you can take to protect yourself and stay healthy:

1. Stay on established trails.
2. Wear light-colored long pants with the legs tucked into your socks, and a long-sleeved shirt (the light color helps you spot any ticks).
3. Use a tick repellent containing Permethrin (sold as Permatone) to *pretreat* your clothes; do not spray on exposed skin or on clothes you are currently wearing.
4. Upon returning to the trailhead, inspect clothing for ticks.
5. Upon returning home, shake and brush all clothes outside; then wash them.
6. Shower and inspect yourself for ticks; use a magnifying glass to check any suspicious dark spots or bumps (ticks have legs).

Unlike wood ticks, which are large enough to be easily visible, the tick that carries Lyme disease, called a deer tick, is tiny—about the size of a pinhead. If you find a tick attached, remove it using a pair of tweezers as follows: grasp the tick as close to your skin as possible and then gently rotate it out; be careful not to squeeze the tick, as this may cause it to inject you with the disease-causing spirochete. Clean the bite area, apply antiseptic, and see a doctor. Current research indicates that 200 milligrams of doxycycline, if taken within 72 hours of a tick bite, will prevent Lyme disease in an adult.

POISON IVY

Poison ivy on the Cape and Islands grows as both a ground cover and a climbing vine, but the rule for recognizing and avoiding it is the same: "leaflets three, let it be." All parts of the plant contain urushiol, the oil that causes severe itching, redness, swelling, and then blisters in sensitive people. The best way to protect yourself is to stay on established trails and wear long pants and a long-sleeved shirt. Over-the-counter barrier skin creams may be helpful. When you get home, wash anything that came in contact with poison ivy, including yourself, your gear and clothing, and your pet; be careful not to contaminate household items.

If your bare skin contacts poison ivy, washing immediately may help prevent or reduce the extent of the rash. If you do contract a rash from poison ivy—this may happen within 12 to 48 hours—do not scratch it, as this could cause infection. Wash and dry the rash thoroughly, and then apply calamine lotion. Cool showers, or soaking in a lukewarm oatmeal or baking-soda solution may reduce itching and dry blisters. Medications, including prescription cortisone, may be indicated; if you have had severe reactions in the past and know you have just been exposed, see your doctor.

BITING INSECTS

Mosquitoes, biting midges, greenheads, deer flies—yikes! Anyone who has spent time on the Cape and Islands during the summer months has probably waged a constant battle with biting insects. Fortunately, many of the same measures recommended to block ticks

INTRODUCTION

and poison ivy—long pants and a long-sleeved shirt—will also help fend off bothersome bitters, including the mosquitoes that cause West Nile virus, which made its first appearance on Cape Cod during the summer of 2005.

Some folks swear by various sprays and lotions, including repellents containing DEET, and more recently Picaridin, whereas others favor "bug-proof" clothing, but the bottom line is this: cover up, use a repellent, or cower.

In addition to appropriate attire, route choice, season, time of day, and wind speed all affect how bad the bugs will be. Here are some examples:

Mosquitoes are most bothersome in shady areas and also at dawn and dusk; season is generally June through August, although they are also here in May and September.

Biting midges, or no-see-ums, are most bothersome around salt water when the air is still; season is generally early to midsummer.

Greenhead flies, related to horse flies, are most bothersome in and near salt marshes, especially when the air is still or the wind is coming from the land; season is generally July and August.

Deer flies, also related to horseflies, are found in upland areas; season is generally July and August.

HUNTING

Many of the walks in this book are in areas where hunting is allowed in season, generally fall and winter. Whereas waterfowl hunting does not usually pose a threat to woodland walkers, deer hunting definitely does. During hunting season, if you visit areas where hunting is allowed, be sure to wear highly visible clothing (for example an orange cap and vest), stay on marked trails, and leash your pet (where pets are allowed).

You can find a complete schedule of Massachusetts hunting seasons for various animals, along with other information, at **www.mass.gov/dfwele/dfw/dfwrec.htm#HUNT.** (Note that hunting is not allowed on Sundays.) In addition, the Trail Use section of the **At-a-Glance Information** for each walk states whether hunting is allowed or not. Finally, Appendix A has a list of walks in areas where hunting is *not* allowed.

SUN PROTECTION

Although nearly everyone enjoys a bright, sunny day, the harmful effects of prolonged exposure to the sun's ultraviolet (UV) rays are well known—and these rays are present on cloudy days as well. The **At-a-Glance Information** for each walk (see page 18) tells you the route's sun exposure: most of the walks in this book have full or partial exposure. Sun protection involves both physical and chemical barriers—clothing, hat, and sunscreen. In recent years, manufacturers of outdoor clothing have become sun-savvy, and today you can find shirts, pants, and hats with special fabrics or treatments to fend of UV rays. So proper attire, combined with liberal and frequent application of sunscreen (30 SPF or above) to any exposed skin will help you stay sun-safe.

WATER

If you bring only one thing along on your walk (aside from this book), make it water. Very few of the trailheads provide water, and there is no potable water on any of the

INTRODUCTION

routes. The combination of warm temperatures and high humidity found on the Cape and Islands during the summer makes it necessary to keep yourself well hydrated before, during, and after your walk. Even during the cooler months, it is a good idea to carry water to prevent dehydration. Remember, children and pets need water too. What's more, you'll find it nearly impossible to choke down an energy bar or other snack without water. How much water is enough? Figure on about one quart per person on all but the longest walks in this book; for those trips, two quarts is recommended.

FIRST-AID KIT

The most important first-aid item is one you have with you at all times—it is located between your ears. A little common sense will help you avoid situations that require first aid. For example:

1. Know your physical limitations and those of your companions; don't try to go too far too fast, or without proper conditioning.
2. Wear appropriate clothing and footwear.
3. Stay on the trail.
4. Never approach or try to handle wildlife.
5. Stay well hydrated and nourished; avoid fatigue.
6. Pay attention to the weather, especially the threat of lightning and/or high winds, which may topple trees.

Most of the walks in this book take you only an hour or two from the trailhead, so if you keep a well-stocked first-aid kit in your car (and you should), you don't need to carry more than a few basic items in your pack. These might include bandages, gauze pads, waterproof tape, waterless hand cleaner or antibacterial wipes, pills for pain and/or inflammation (aspirin, acetaminophen, ibuprofen, etc.), and any medicine you may need for specific health conditions (such as a severe allergic reaction to bee stings).

WALKING WITH CHILDREN

Walking with children presents special challenges, but it also brings great rewards. Seeing the natural world through a child's eyes is a great way to relearn why going for a walk in the woods is such a treat. Remember that children may not be as goal-oriented as you are, so be prepared to scale back your expectations, such as reaching a certain destination, or completing a particular route. Children love to dawdle, to look at things, and to ask lots of questions; they may be more concerned with the *process* of walking than the end result.

Various contraptions, including backpack-style child carriers and strollers designed for trail use, allow children too young to walk (or walk very far) to accompany adults on their outings. Even if the children are proficient walkers, it's a good idea to start out with walks graded as "Easy" in the **At-a-Glance Information** (see page 16). No matter what their age, children need protection from ticks, poison ivy, biting insects, and the sun— just like adults do. Children also need proper footwear, clothing, water, and snacks.

INTRODUCTION

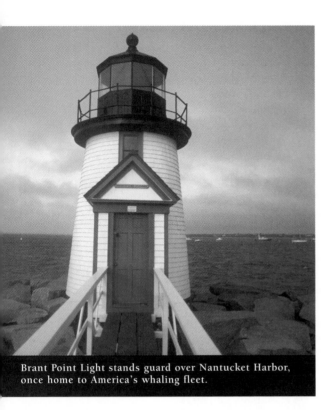

Brant Point Light stands guard over Nantucket Harbor, once home to America's whaling fleet.

A list of walks recommended for children is in Appendix A. Because most of the trailheads on the Cape and Islands have no facilities, this list contains only easy walks that begin at a nature center or other venue where water and restrooms are available. Self-guided nature walks, especially ones that have descriptive brochures, are particularly fun for children (and adults too), because they usually provide lots of things to look at and learn about along the way.

TRAIL ETIQUETTE

Many of the open spaces on the Cape and Islands have multiuse trails—that is, in addition to walking and hiking they are used for jogging, dog walking, bicycling, and (rarely) horseback riding. Unlike the complex rules of sailing, determining right-of-way on a multiuse trail is simple: travelers on foot yield to equestrians, bicyclists yield to everyone. Also simple is the code of behavior that ensures everyone, now and in the future, will be able to enjoy the trails: take only photographs, leave only footprints, walk only on designated trails, and respect private property.

DOGS

Many people enjoy walking with their dogs, and there is no doubt the dogs enjoy it too. However, before bringing your dog on the trail, here are some things to consider:

• Are dogs allowed? The Trail Use section of the **At-a-Glance Information** for each walk states whether dogs are allowed on the route as described. A list of walks where dogs are *not* allowed on the route as described is in Appendix A.

• Where dogs are allowed, they generally must be leashed; in a few areas, dogs are allowed under *immediate* voice command. This means the dog will instantly stop what it is doing, e.g., chasing a squirrel, and return to its owner. There are few things as frightening on the trail as having a large, barking dog approaching, with its owner 100 feet away yelling "I said COME!" or, perhaps worse, "It's OK; he's friendly."

INTRODUCTION

- Where dogs are allowed, it is always required that you clean up after your pet.
- Ticks and poison ivy are just about everywhere on the Cape and Islands, and dogs are almost certain to come into contact with them on the trail.
- Coyotes, skunks, and raccoons—all potentially hazardous to your pet—inhabit many of the open spaces on the Cape and Islands.
- Rabies is now present in parts of Cape Cod.
- Many of the walks in this book pass through critical wildlife habitat, where a variety of animals live, feed, rest, raise young, or pass through on migration. Dogs, if left to run free, may chase, threaten, or disturb wildlife.

▶ HOW TO USE THIS BOOK

This book is organized geographically by region, generally following the organization of Kim Grant's *Cape Cod, Martha's Vineyard, & Nantucket: An Explorer's Guide*. These regions are: Upper Cape, Mid-Cape, Lower Cape, Outer Cape, Martha's Vineyard, and Nantucket.

Within these regions are the Cape's 15 towns: Bourne, Sandwich, Falmouth, Mashpee (Upper Cape); Barnstable, Hyannis, Yarmouth, Dennis (Mid-Cape); Brewster, Harwich, Chatham, Orleans (Lower Cape); and Eastham, Wellfleet, Truro, Provincetown (Outer Cape). Each town may have several villages; for example, the Town of Barnstable has a village named Barnstable, along with the villages of West Barnstable, Hyannis, and Hyannisport. (Barnstable is also the name of the county that covers Cape Cod.)

Note: The terms *upper* and *lower* do not refer to positions on the map, but rather to distance from the mainland. Whether this terminology follows nautical usage—sailing upwind or downwind, longitude increasing as one travels westward—or was done intentionally to confuse the tourists, no one knows for sure.

Martha's Vineyard is represented in this book by five towns: Chilmark, Edgartown (which contains Chappaquiddick Island), Oak Bluffs, Tisbury, and West Tisbury. A sixth town, Aquinnah (formerly Gay Head), is home to many of the island's Wampanoag people and is also the site of the dramatic Gay Head cliffs, but has only a very small amount of public land with walking trails. Nantucket has a central town, also named Nantucket, and a handful of small villages.

The route description for each walk in this book is preceded by concise, helpful info, including the **Walk Area**, the **Walk Name, At-a-Glance Information, Health Stats,** a **Walk Summary,** and **Directions to Trailhead.** For the Cape and the Vineyard, the **Walk Area** refers to the town and the open space where the walk is located. For Nantucket (which is a single town), only the name of the open space is given. The **Walk Name** is generally the author's creation, sometimes whimsical, to characterize the walk.

The **At-a-Glance Information** contains all the vital statistics pertaining to the walk, as follows:

DISTANCE An estimate of the total round-trip distance for the walk, done exactly as described. Estimates are based on pedometer measurements, computer mapping, agency maps, and GPS data.

INTRODUCTION

TYPE OF WALK This describes the shape of the route, which may be either **loop, out-and-back,** or **balloon** (a loop with an out-and-back leg).

DIFFICULTY A subjective estimate of the walk's difficulty, as follows: 2 miles or less and flat, **easy;** between one and five miles with some hills, **moderate;** more than 5 miles, difficult. Within the route description, steepness is indicated by the words "gentle," "moderate," and "steep." A gentle ascent/descent is barely noticeable; a moderate ascent/descent usually requires a change of pace and/or stride length; a steep ascent/descent involves huffing and puffing on the way up, and caution on the way down.

TIME TO WALK An estimated time range, based on the author's average speed of two miles per hour (including stops for rest, snacks, nature study, photography) to complete the walk, done exactly as described.

MAPS The map produced by the agency administering the open space (if available), followed by the appropriate USGS 7.5 minute quadrangle map. Maps for many of the walks described in this book are available only from the agencies administering the open spaces; some are available to download from agency Web sites (see Appendix C). A few trailheads have map holders, but these may be empty. If there is a visitor center (see Facilities, below), a map is usually available there. *Note:* When a map is referred to in the route description, it is always the agency map unless otherwise stated.

SCENERY A brief list of the major habitats seen from the route.

EXPOSURE TO SUN Described as **none, partial,** or **full,** the amount of solar exposure on the route, done exactly as described.

TRAIL TRAFFIC An estimate of the amount of trail traffic during July and August on *any* segment of the described route, given as **light, moderate,** or **heavy.**

TRAIL SURFACE(S) A description of the trail surface, usually either **dirt, sand, pavement,** or some combination.

TRAILS OPEN The trails in this book are generally open all year, but some areas may have restrictions during hunting season. Hours are usually sunrise to sunset, but some areas have specific opening and closing times, and these may vary depending on the season. For detailed information about a specific area, look under **Maps** (see above) to find the overseeing agency, and then check that agency's Web site, listed in Appendix C.

FEES/PASSES A few walks in this book visit areas that require an entrance fee, which is usually either reduced or waived for members of the organization overseeing the area, such as the Massachusetts Audubon Society or The Trustees of Reservations.

FACILITIES A list of the facilities found at or near the trailhead, such as **restrooms, toilet (no running water), water, visitor/nature center,** or **phone.** *Note:* Most areas described in this book have no facilities, and those that do usually have them open only during the summer season.

INTRODUCTION

TRAIL USE Indicates if the route as described is open to bicycles, dogs, and/or hunting.

Also preceding each of the route descriptions are **Health Stats,** which consist of the **number of steps** and the **estimated calories burned.** Number of steps is an approximation derived from the walk's total distance, based on the author's average stride length of 28 inches; thus, 1 mile equals approximately 2,250 steps. The estimated calories burned is an approximation based on the author's weight of 155 pounds; therefore, it will take approximately 21 steps for a 155-pound walker to burn 1 calorie (1 mile will burn approximately 107 calories).

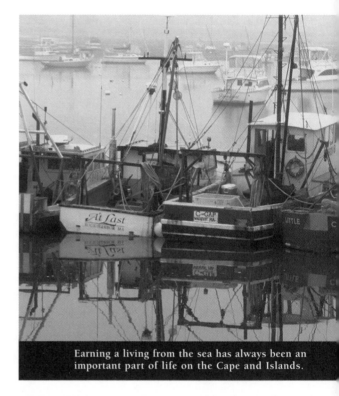

Earning a living from the sea has always been an important part of life on the Cape and Islands.

The **Walk Summary** gives readers a descriptive snapshot of what the walk is like, including any notable features of human or natural history. **Directions to Trailhead** provides precise driving directions from the nearest major roadway to the parking area that serves the trailhead. (Road and street names are from the Official Arrow™ street atlas for Cape Cod, Martha's Vineyard, and Nantucket; local names, if different, are in parentheses.) Then the location of the trailhead is given by compass direction, i.e. "The trailhead is on the west side of the parking area." *Note:* Martha's Vineyard and Nantucket have mass-transit options to reach some of the trailheads described in this book (see Appendix C for Martha's Vineyard Transit Authority, Nantucket Regional Transit Authority). Bicycling on these islands is also a car-free way to reach trailheads, but be sure to lock your bike at the trailhead.

The **Description** is text designed to lead readers from the trailhead and back again following a specific route. The Description includes all junctions and instructions on what to do when reaching them, i.e., continue straight or turn left or right. The text may also mention trail names, signage (if present), landscape features, and other items of interest.

For each walk, most aspects of natural history are presented in the **Flora Sidebar** and the **Fauna Sidebar.** These are not complete listings of all species present; rather

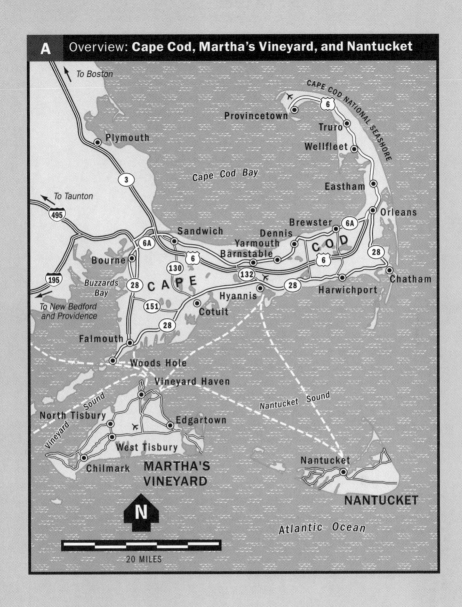

To Boston

Provincetown

CAPE COD NATIONAL SEASHORE

6

Truro

Wellfleet

Plymouth

Cape Cod Bay

3

Eastham

To Taunton

495

Orleans

Brewster 6A

Sandwich

Dennis

CO D

Yarmouth

Bourne

6A

6

Barnstable

6

28

Buzzards
Bay

195

28

C A P E

130

132

28

Chatham

To New Bedford
and Providence

151

Hyannis

Cotuit

28

Harwichport

Falmouth

28

Woods Hole

Vineyard Haven

Nantucket Sound

North Tisbury

Sound

Vineyard

Edgartown

West Tisbury

Nantucket

Chilmark **MARTHA'S
VINEYARD**

NANTUCKET

N

Atlantic Ocean

20 MILES

they are observations the author made on the day(s) he visited the area, combined in some cases with listings provided by the overseeing agency or other reliable source.

Finally, the book contains three **Appendixes. Appendix A** groups walks by various criteria, including difficulty, whether dogs and/or hunting are allowed, best birding walks, best nature walks, best off-season walks, best scenic vistas, best walks with children, and best wildflowers. **Appendix B** is a list of recommended reading. **Appendix C** is a list of information sources—relevant government agencies, nonprofit organizations, businesses, and private groups—with their phone numbers and URLs.

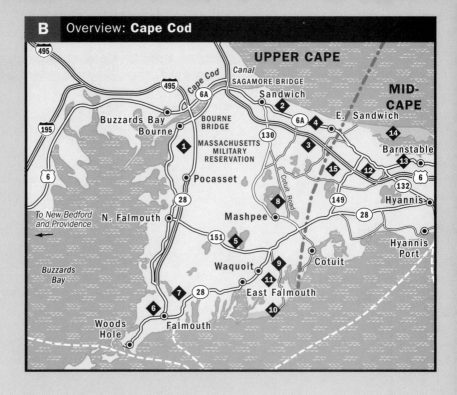

CAPE COD: UPPER CAPE

1 Town Forest Tour: *Bourne, Four Ponds Conservation Area*
2 Boiling Springs Pond: *Sandwich, Briar Patch Conservation Area*
3 Moraine Ramble: *Sandwich, Maple Swamp Conservation Lands*
4 Scorton Creek Marsh: *Sandwich, Murkwood Conservation Area*
5 Grassy Pond: *Falmouth, Ashumet Holly Wildlife Sanctuary (Mass Audubon)*
6 Punch Bowl: *Falmouth, Beebe Woods*
7 Long Pond: *Falmouth, Falmouth Town Forest*
8 Two-Pond Ramble: *Mashpee, Lowell Holly Reservation*
9 West Side Trek: *Mashpee, Mashpee River Woodlands*
10 Great Flat Pond Trail: *Mashpee, South Cape Beach State Park*
11 Pine Barrens: *Mashpee, South Mashpee Pine Barrens Conservation Area*

CAPE COD: MID-CAPE

12 East Side Ramble: *Barnstable, Bridge Creek Conservation Area*
13 Forest Foray: *Barnstable, Old Jail Lane Conservation Area*
14 Great Marshes to Cape Cod Bay: *Barnstable, Sandy Neck*
15 Moraine Trek: *Barnstable, West Barnstable Conservation Area*
16 Grand Traverse: *Yarmouth, Callery-Darling Conservation Area*
17 Nature Trail: *Yarmouth, Historical Society of Old Yarmouth*
18 Shoreline Loop: *Dennis, Crowes Pasture*
19 Bass River Ramble: *Dennis, Indian Lands Conservation Area*

CAPE COD: LOWER CAPE

20 John Wing Trail: *Brewster, Cape Cod Museum of Natural History*
21 Cliff and Little Cliff Ponds: *Brewster, Nickerson State Park*
22 Silas Road: *Brewster, Nickerson State Park*
23 Calf Field Pond: *Brewster, Punkhorn Parklands*
24 Eagle Point: *Brewster, Punkhorn Parklands*
25 Grand Tour: *Brewster, Punkhorn Parklands*
26 Herring River: *Harwich, Bells Neck Road Conservation Area*
27 Kettle Pond Ramble: *Harwich, Hawksnest State Park*
28 Morris Island Trail: *Chatham, Monomoy National Wildlife Refuge*
29 Kent's Point: *Orleans, Kent's Point Conservation Area*
30 Bayside Stroll: *Orleans, Paw Wah Pond Conservation Area*

CAPE COD: OUTER CAPE

31 Nauset Marsh Trail and Coast Guard Beach: *Eastham, Cape Cod National Seashore*
32 Red Maple Swamp and Fort Hill: *Eastham, Cape Cod National Seashore*
33 Atlantic White Cedar Swamp Trail: *Wellfleet, Cape Cod National Seashore*
34 Great Island Trail: *Wellfleet, Cape Cod National Seashore*
35 Wellfleet and Truro Ponds: *Wellfleet, Cape Cod National Seashore*
36 Bay View Trail and Fresh Brook Pathway: *Wellfleet, Wellfleet Bay Wildlife Sanctuary (Mass Audubon)*
37 Goose Pond Trail: *Wellfleet, Wellfleet Bay Wildlife Sanctuary (Mass Audubon)*
38 Bearberry Hill and Bog House: *Truro, Cape Cod National Seashore, North Pamet Area*

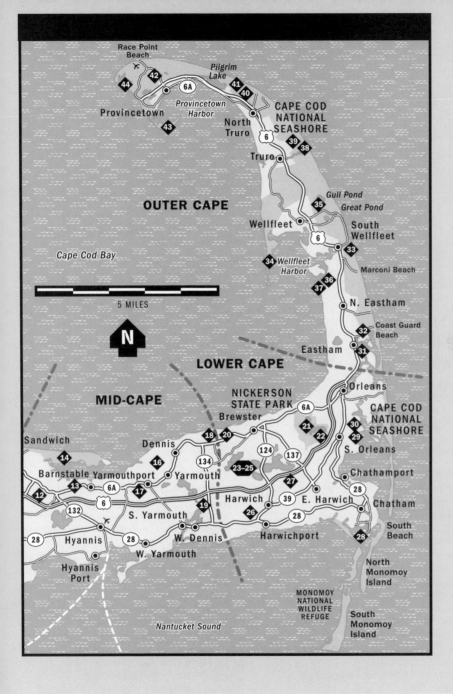

Race Point
Beach
Pilgrim
Lake
44 42 6A 41 40
CAPE COD
Provincetown Provincetown NATIONAL
Harbor North SEASHORE
43 Truro 6
39 38
Truro
OUTER CAPE Gull Pond
35 Great Pond
Wellfleet South
Cape Cod Bay 6 Wellfleet
33
34 Wellfleet
Harbor Marconi Beach
5 MILES 36
37 N. Eastham

N

Coast Guard
32 Beach
Eastham 31
LOWER CAPE
Orleans
MID-CAPE NICKERSON
STATE PARK 6A CAPE COD
Brewster NATIONAL
21 30 SEASHORE
18 20 22 29
Sandwich Dennis S. Orleans
124
14 16 134 137 Chathamport
Barnstable Yarmouthport Yarmouth 23-25
13 6A 27 28
12 17 Harwich 39 E. Harwich Chatham
132 6 19
S. Yarmouth 26 28 South
28 28 W. Dennis Harwichport 28 Beach
Hyannis
W. Yarmouth
Hyannis North
Port Monomoy
Island
MONOMOY
NATIONAL
WILDLIFE South
REFUGE Monomoy
Nantucket Sound Island

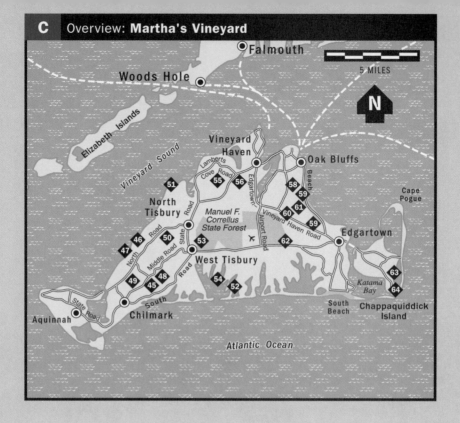

C Overview: **Martha's Vineyard**

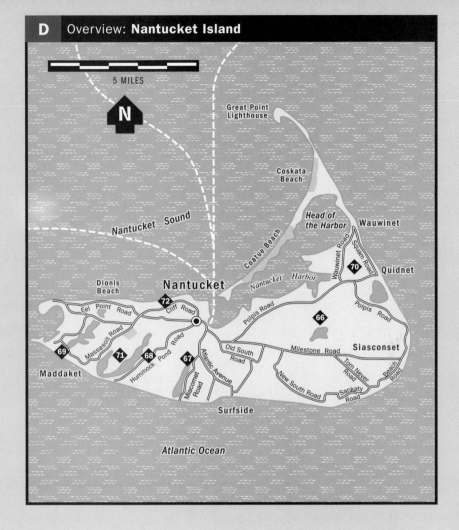

5 MILES

N

Great Point
Lighthouse

Coskata
Beach

Nantucket Sound

Head of
the Harbor   Wauwinet

Coatue Beach

Dionis
Beach

Nantucket

Nantucket Harbor

Quidnet

72

Eel Point Road   Cliff Road

Polpis Road

66

Polpis Road

Siasconset

Massasoit Road

Old South
Road

Milestone Road

69   **71**   **68**   **67**

Hummock Pond Road

Atlantic Avenue

Miacomet Road

New South Road

Tom Never Road

Sankaty Road

Beach Road

Maddaket

Surfside

Atlantic Ocean

NANTUCKET

66 Moorish Delight: *Nantucket, Altar Rock*

67 Miacomet Pond: *Nantucket, Burchell*

68 Forest, Meadow, and Marsh Meander:
Nantucket, Gardner

69 Pond Promenade: *Nantucket, Long Pond*

70 Squam Swamp Interpretive Trail: *Nantucket,
Squam Swamp*

71 Barn and Back: *Nantucket, The Sanford Farm,
Ram Pasture, and The Woods*

72 A Link to the Past: *Nantucket, Tupancy Links*

Cape Cod: Upper Cape

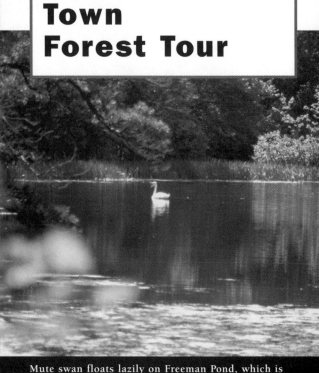
KEY AT-A-GLANCE INFORMATION

GENERAL

DISTANCE 3.6 miles

TYPE OF WALK Balloon

DIFFICULTY Moderate

TIME TO WALK 2–3 hours

MAPS *Four Ponds Walking Trails,* Bourne Conservation Commission; *Pocasset,* USGS

SCENERY Forest, ponds

EXPOSURE TO SUN Partial

TRAIL TRAFFIC Light

TRAIL SURFACE(S) Dirt

TRAILS OPEN All year

FEES/PASSES None

FACILITIES None

TRAIL USE

BICYCLES Allowed only on Pine and Town Forest trails

DOGS Allowed on leash

HUNTING Allowed in season north from Upper Pond to the Town Forest

HEALTH STATS

NUMBER OF STEPS 8,100

ESTIMATED CALORIES BURNED 386

DIRECTIONS TO TRAILHEAD

From Route 28 southbound in Bourne, 3.4 miles south of the Bourne rotary, turn right on Barlows Landing Road, signed for Pocasset and Wings Neck. Go 0.7 miles to a gravel parking area, right.

From Route 28 northbound in Bourne, turn left at the exit signed for Pocasset and Wings Neck, make a U-turn to access Route 28 southbound; then follow the directions above.

The trailhead is on the north side of the parking area.

Mute swan floats lazily on Freeman Pond, which is one pond in Four Ponds Conservation Area.

WALK SUMMARY

Named for the four bodies of water within its boundaries—Shop Pond, Freeman Pond, Upper Pond, and The Basin—this conservation area borders the Bourne Town Forest. The two areas combined provide a 280-acre wooded wonderland, perfect for exploring on foot, that is almost within earshot of busy Route 28. A variety of multiuse dirt roads and trails crisscross the mostly rolling terrain, which hosts a botanically rich array of trees and shrubs.

DESCRIPTION

The initial path that you will take is actually four trails joined as one, which soon diverge. To begin, head north about 100 yards to an information board. The trails are color-coded as follows: Eagle

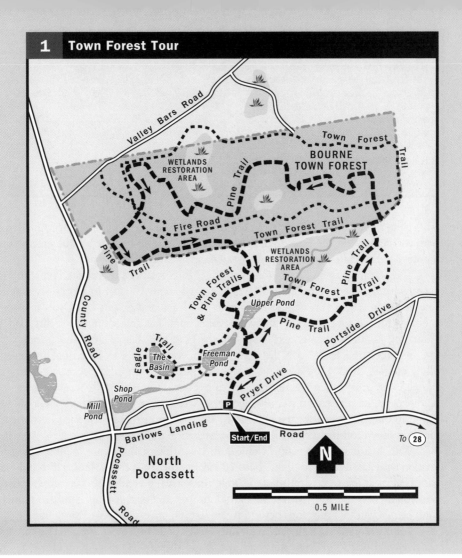

Trail—red; Town Forest Trail—green; Lions Trail—blue; Pine Trail—black.

Veer right onto the Pine Trail, which here is also the Town Forest Trail, and descend through dense forest on a dirt trail carpeted with pine needles. A rest bench is on the left, and Freeman Pond is beyond it, through the trees. The ponds in this conservation area are actually impoundments on a spring-fed brook that, until the early 1800s, flowed freely into the Pocasset River. The impoundments served as a source of power for a nearby iron foundry.

Where the Lions Trail joins from the left, head to the right. Cross a possibly wet area via a short boardwalk and then climb past a rest bench on your right. At the next junction, the Pine Trail splits to begin a loop, and you go

FLORA	FAUNA
Pitch pine, white pine, scrub oak, black oak, white oak, black cherry, red maple, sassafras, and American holly characterize forests on the upper Cape. Shrubs here include sweet pepperbush, lowbush blueberry, black huckleberry, bayberry, swamp azalea, arrowwood, wild raisin, wild rose, dwarf chestnut oak, and hazelnut. Near the ponds grow alder, chokeberry, sheep laurel, and highbush blueberry.	Blue jays, black-capped chickadees, American robins, northern cardinals, woodpeckers, and warblers may be your avian companions. Mute swans, beautiful to look at but considered harmful to other birds by most wildlife experts, may be floating on the ponds, along with ducks.

right. Upper Pond is on your left. Where unsigned trails depart from your route, bypass them and remain on the Pine Trail. A large boulder, left, is evidence of the glacial forces that formed this part of the Cape. A rest bench is nearby on the right.

The winding, rolling trail crosses a ridge, then resumes its roller-coaster ride to a merger with the Town Forest Trail. Veer right and go about 100 feet to a four-way junction. Here you turn left to stay on the Pine Trail. More ups and downs bring you to another meeting with the Town Forest Trail, where you'll angle left and soon meet a dirt road at a T-junction. Jog right, then go left to stay on the Pine Trail, here a single-track trail.

A level stroll leads to a dirt road, which you cross. The Pine Trail resumes its rolling course, curving left at about the 1-mile point to skirt a bog. Atop a ridge, you'll enjoy an easy stroll, then wander parallel to a dirt path on your left. Steering away from the dirt path, soon cross a dirt-and-gravel road and begin a moderate climb. Gaining elevation, in one place steeply, pass a clearing on your right that is screened from view by trees but shown on the map as a wetland restoration area.

With just enough elevation changes to keep things interesting, ramble along to a junction with a trail that goes right about 100 feet to the Town Forest Trail, a dirt-and-gravel road. Here bear left to stay on the Pine Trail. After a steep climb puts you atop a plateau, soon you'll cross the Town Forest Trail at a four-way junction. A long, gentle-to-moderate climb carries you to a ridgetop; beyond it you'll again cross the Town Forest Trail.

Rolling along, curve sharply right and meet the Town Forest Trail, here a dirt road, at a five-way junction. Cross the road and angle slightly left to stay on the Pine Trail, joined here by part of the Town Forest Trail. You'll gain a ridgetop, run it for a while, drop to a low area at about 3 miles, and then climb steeply. Losing the hard-won altitude, pass a trail on your right; then turn left on a wide dirt path. At a T-junction with a dirt road, turn left again and descend on a gentle grade. At the next junction, veer right onto a dirt road beside Upper Pond, which is left.

When you reach a junction with the Lions Trail, turn left, pass a rest bench, and walk across a concrete bridge followed by a wooden bridge, between Upper and Freeman ponds. This is a lovely spot, with views of both ponds and a botanically rich array of vegetation. Once across the bridges, bear right at a fork with an unsigned trail. At the next junction, close the loop with the Pine Trail. From here, go straight and retrace your route to the parking area, remembering to bear left at the next junction.

Boiling Springs Pond

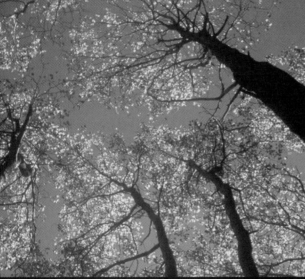

Pines, oaks, red maples, and hickories are some of the trees that grace this lovely conservation area.

WALK SUMMARY

This circuit of Boiling Springs Pond, also called Smiling Pool, explores an area beloved by Sandwich native Thornton W. Burgess (1874–1965), creator of Peter Rabbit and other memorable characters in his many books for children. The wooded trails here traverse slopes shaded by a variety of tall trees, including magnificent white pines. The pond itself, mostly hidden from view, is bordered by a swamp, whose vegetation provides a colorful display in fall.

The Green Briar Nature Center and Jam Kitchen, operated by the Thornton W. Burgess Society, sit on the pond's north shore. The nature center features flora and fauna displays, a wildflower garden, and the Robert S. Swain Natural History Library. The Jam Kitchen, established in 1903 by

KEY AT-A-GLANCE INFORMATION

GENERAL

DISTANCE 1.3 miles

TYPE OF WALK Loop

DIFFICULTY Easy

TIME TO WALK 1 hour or less

MAPS Trail map available at nature center; *Sandwich*, USGS

SCENERY Forest, pond

EXPOSURE TO SUN Partial

TRAIL TRAFFIC Moderate

TRAIL SURFACE(S) Dirt, paved

TRAILS OPEN All year

FEES/PASSES None

FACILITIES None at the trailhead; restrooms and picnic tables at the nature center

TRAIL USE

BICYCLES Not allowed

DOGS Allowed on leash May 1– August 31; leashed or under voice control September 1–April 30

HUNTING Allowed in season

HEALTH STATS

NUMBER OF STEPS 2,925

ESTIMATED CALORIES BURNED 139

DIRECTIONS TO TRAILHEAD

From the intersection of Route 6A and Discovery Hill Road in Sandwich, take Discovery Hill Road southeast several hundred feet to a large dirt parking area, right. The trailhead is on the northwest corner of the parking area.

Note: The entrance to the Green Briar Nature Center is several hundred feet farther southeast on Discovery Hill Road; the parking area there is small and often filled in summer.

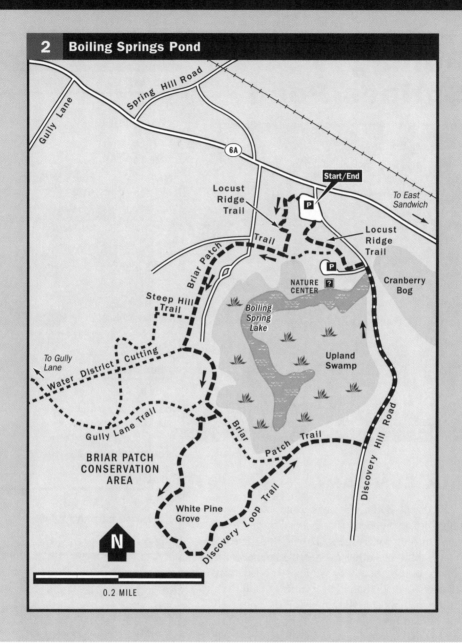

2 Boiling Springs Pond

Ida Putnam, still makes jams and jellies the old-fashioned way and functions as a living museum.

Hours for the nature center and the Jam Kitchen: April through December, Monday through Saturday, 10 a.m. to 4 p.m., Sunday, 1 to 4 p.m.; January through March, Tuesday through Saturday, 10 a.m. to 4 p.m. Admission to the nature center and the Jam Kitchen is by donation. The Thornton W. Burgess Museum is located on Shawme Pond in Sandwich at 4 Water Street (Route 130).

DESCRIPTION

From the trailhead, follow the single-track Locust Ridge Trail through dense underbrush, passing a seasonal wetland, right. The trail swings left to a T-junction, where a short trail to the nature center joins from the left. Here get on the Briar Patch Trail by turning right. Climb gently to cross a paved road; then enjoy a mostly level traverse across a forested hillside. A watershed (no trespassing) is behind a fence, left.

Now the Steep Hill Trail departs uphill to the right. Just ahead is a fork. Stay left and descend moderately, walking through a gap in a stone wall. Soon you pass a trail, left, into the watershed. Bear right and go several hundred yards to a junction. Turn left and skirt the swamp bordering Boiling Springs Pond. At the next junction, turn right and stroll past a rest bench to a fork. Here the Gully Lane Trail goes right, and the Discovery Loop Trail (signed DISCOVERY HILL LOOP) goes left.

Bear left and climb a moderate but short pitch to a peaceful white-pine grove, where the ground may be carpeted with delicate needles in bunches of five, and littered with long, cylindrical cones. Rest benches along the way offer quiet spots for contemplation. The trail bends left and descends gently to meet the Briar Patch Trail, which joins from the left. Go straight at the next junction, pass a rest bench, and soon meet paved Discovery Hill Road.

Turn left and walk along the road shoulder, facing traffic. Your first good view of the picturesque pond is left. A cranberry bog is right, across the road. Soon you reach the entrance road for the nature center, left (certainly worth a visit if open). Go left and find the trailhead for the Locust Ridge Trail, which is beside a large sign for the nature center, on the right (north) side of the entrance road. The trail climbs moderately through stands of black locust, crosses a ridge, and then winds downhill to the south side of the parking area.

GENERAL

DISTANCE 2.5 miles

TYPE OF WALK Balloon

DIFFICULTY Moderate

TIME TO WALK 1–2 hours

MAPS *Town of Sandwich Conservation and Recreation Land,* Sandwich Environmental Task Force; *Sandwich,* USGS

SCENERY Forest

EXPOSURE TO SUN None

TRAIL TRAFFIC Light

TRAIL SURFACE(S) Dirt

TRAILS OPEN All year

FEES/PASSES None

FACILITIES None

TRAIL USE

BICYCLES Not allowed on single-track trails, including part of this route

DOGS Allowed on leash May 1–August 31; leashed or under voice control September 1–April 30

HUNTING Allowed in season

HEALTH STATS

NUMBER OF STEPS 5,625

ESTIMATED CALORIES BURNED 268

DIRECTIONS TO TRAILHEAD

From Route 6 westbound in Sandwich, take Exit 4, go left (south) on Chase Road 0.1 mile, and turn right on Service Road. Go 1.1 mile to a paved parking area, left.

From Route 6 eastbound in Sandwich, take Exit 3, turn right on Quaker Meetinghouse Road; then turn immediately left on Service Road. Go 1.1 mile to a paved parking area, right.

The trailhead is on the south side of the parking area at a green gate.

Moraine Ramble

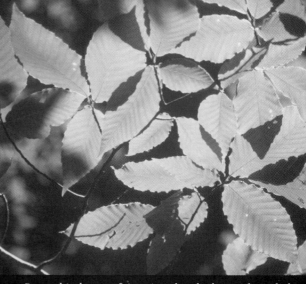

Paper-thin leaves of American beech glow with sunlight in a dark forest.

WALK SUMMARY

The Cape's glacial origins are to thank for this leg-stretching ramble along the Sandwich moraine. A secluded picnic table with a glancing view of Cape Cod Bay, soon perhaps to be lost to the fast-growing forest, rewards your uphill efforts.

DESCRIPTION

From the trailhead, follow a dirt road into a forest of mostly pine and oak. After 100 yards or so, meet another trail from the parking area, joining sharply from the right. Stay right at an upcoming fork; there is a white blaze on a pine tree to the left of the trail. In places trails lead off into the woods, but ignore them to stay on the described route. Follow a dirt road gently downhill, passing a seasonal wetland on your right. A large boulder also on the right

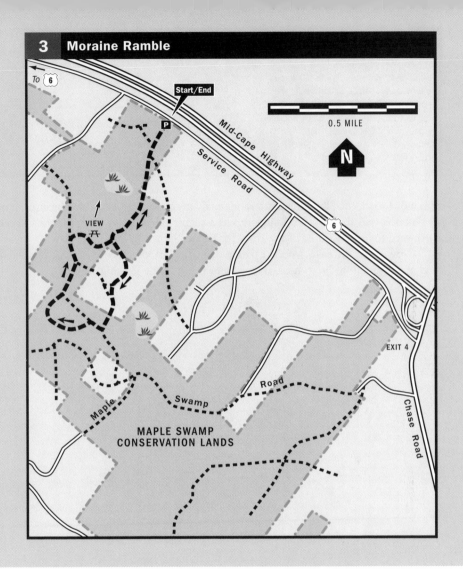

To 6

Start/End

P

Mid-Cape Highway

Service Road

0.5 MILE

N

6

VIEW

EXIT 4

Maple

Swamp

Road

Chase Road

**MAPLE SWAMP
CONSERVATION LANDS**

evidences the Cape's glacial past, particularly the moraine that is responsible for the hilly terrain found here.

Now on a gentle and then moderate climb, the rocky road twists its way to a high point, then begins to descend. Stay on the road through junctions with several trails until you meet a fork. Bear left and almost immediately merge with another dirt road, which rises on a gentle grade. Soon leave the road and turn right onto a trail that climbs steeply to a fork (the branches rejoin after about a quarter mile).

Bear left and follow the trail as it curves right and descends. Meet the right-hand branch of the previous fork and angle slightly left. At a T-junction

FLORA	FAUNA
The forest here consists mostly of pitch pine, white pine, black oak, white oak, black cherry, red maple, hickory, sassafras, shadbush, and American beech. Shrubs growing beside the route include arrowwood, black huckleberry, highbush blueberry, sweet pepperbush, swamp azalea, and partridgeberry. Asters and goldenrods add color in fall.	Chickadees and blue jays are among the songbirds you might see and hear.

with a dirt road, turn left and climb moderately over rough ground. Now bear right on a single-track trail that follows a ridgetop to a picnic table. From here, the view extends northward to Cape Cod Bay (trees may have since grown to block the view).

Now enjoy an easy, wooded jaunt, then drop moderately to meet a familiar dirt road at a T-junction. From here, retrace your route to the parking area.

Scorton Creek Marsh

 KEY AT-A-GLANCE INFORMATION

GENERAL

DISTANCE 1.2 miles

TYPE OF WALK Balloon

DIFFICULTY Easy

TIME TO WALK 1 hour or less

MAPS *Town of Sandwich Conservation and Recreation Land*, Sandwich Environmental Task Force; *Sandwich*, USGS

SCENERY Forest, salt marsh

EXPOSURE TO SUN None

TRAIL TRAFFIC Light

TRAIL SURFACE(S) Dirt

TRAILS OPEN All year

FEES/PASSES None

FACILITIES None

TRAIL USE

BICYCLES Not allowed

DOGS Allowed on leash May 1– August 31; leashed or under voice control September 1–April 30

HUNTING Allowed in season

HEALTH STATS

NUMBER OF STEPS 2,700

ESTIMATED CALORIES BURNED 129

DIRECTIONS TO TRAILHEAD

From the intersection of Route 6A and Quaker Meetinghouse Road in East Sandwich, take Route 6A southeast 1.3 miles to a parking area, left. The trailhead is on the northwest corner of the parking area.

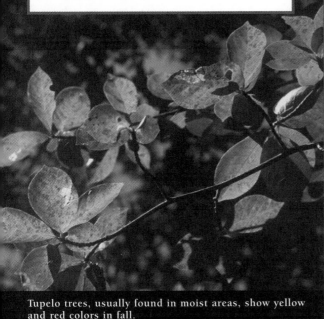

Tupelo trees, usually found in moist areas, show yellow and red colors in fall.

WALK SUMMARY

This short and easy walk explores a beautiful woodland just north of Route 6A and adjacent to Scorton Creek. The creek is bordered by an extensive salt marsh, and views of the marsh are available from the trail. Closely packed houses along East Sandwich Beach can be glimpsed in the distance, offering a reason, if one is needed, to preserve tracts of open space.

DESCRIPTION

Leaving busy Route 6A behind, follow a level trail through the woods to a junction that marks the returning end of a loop. Go straight, cross a plank bridge over a ditch, and reach a rest bench with a view of a salt marsh that borders Scorton Creek, which flows into Cape Cod Bay. Now the trail

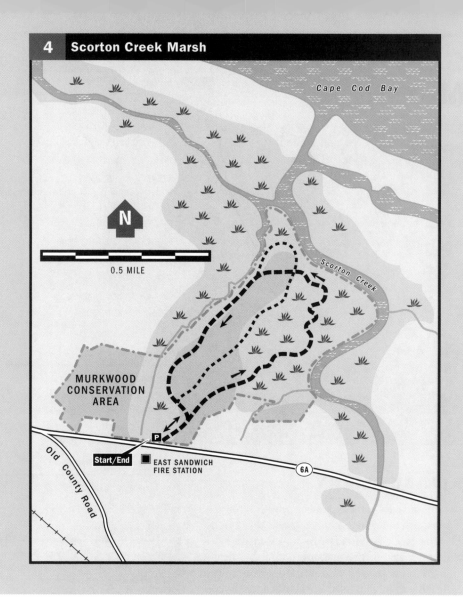

bends left and traverses a junglelike area of twisted pines and formidable ferns. Curve away from the marsh and reach a fork—the right-hand branch leads to a bench overlooking the marsh.

Bear left at the fork and pass a veritable fern garden. Ropy vines of poison ivy twine their way skyward with help from a tree trunk. Roots cross the trail, waiting to trip the unwary walker. With a wet area on the left, cross another plank bridge. Soon swing left and cross a ditch via a long bridge. After closing the loop, veer right and retrace your route to the parking area.

FLORA

This small conservation area is rich in plant life. Trees here include pitch pine, black oak, white oak, black cherry, red maple, eastern red cedar, American holly, and tupelo. The dense understory consists mostly of arrow- wood, bayberry, highbush blueberry, sheep laurel, and greenbrier. Fall colors are provided by the tupelos, in concert with goldenrods, asters, and poison ivy.

FAUNA

Blue jays and American crows, both formida- ble vocalists, may be heard and seen here.

KEY AT-A-GLANCE INFORMATION

GENERAL

DISTANCE 1.1 mile

TYPE OF WALK Balloon

DIFFICULTY Easy

TIME TO WALK 1 hour or less

MAPS *Ashumet Holly Wildlife Sanctuary,* Massachusetts Audubon Society; *Falmouth,* USGS

SCENERY Fields, forest, pond

EXPOSURE TO SUN Partial

TRAIL TRAFFIC Moderate

TRAIL SURFACE(S) Dirt, mowed grass

TRAILS OPEN All year

FEES/PASSES None for Massachusetts Audubon Society members; small fee for nonmembers

FACILITIES Picnic tables

TRAIL USE

BICYCLES Not allowed

DOGS Not allowed

HUNTING Not allowed

HEALTH STATS

NUMBER OF STEPS 2,475

ESTIMATED CALORIES BURNED 118

DIRECTIONS TO TRAILHEAD

From the intersection of Route 28 and Route 151 in North Falmouth, take Route 151 southeast 3.9 miles to Currier Road. Turn left, go 0.1 mile to Ashumet Road, turn right, and then turn immediately left into a parking area.

From the intersection of Route 28 and Route 151 at the Mashpee rotary, take Route 151 west 2.7 miles to Currier Road. Turn right, and then follow the directions above.

The trailhead is located on the north side of the parking area, at an orange metal gate.

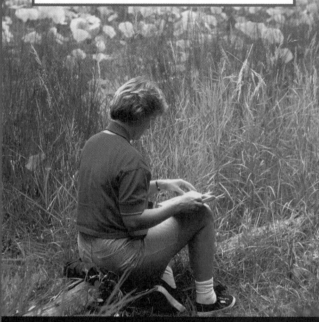

Grassy Pond

This Massachusetts Audubon sanctuary is a great place to learn about native plants.

WALK SUMMARY

This easy jaunt around Grassy Pond has something for everyone. Plant enthusiasts will enjoy the fine collection of native and nonnative trees and shrubs, the variety of forest, meadow, and wetland wildflowers, some quite rare, and, of course, the magnificent holly trees, which give this Massachusetts Audubon Society sanctuary its name. Birders will enjoy watching the aerial antics of a barn swallow colony housed in an old barn near the trailhead. The gentle nature of the well-maintained trails, termed "accessible by wheelchair" in a sanctuary pamphlet, will appeal to families with children. Some of the trail junctions have numbered markers, and all trails are well signed.

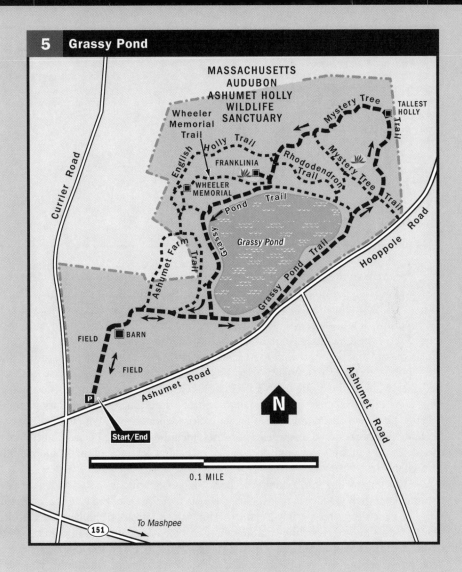

5 Grassy Pond

MASSACHUSETTS
AUDUBON
ASHUMET HOLLY
WILDLIFE
SANCTUARY

Wheeler
Memorial
Trail

Mystery Tree Trail

TALLEST
HOLLY

English Holly Trail

FRANKLINIA

Rhododendron Trail

Mystery Tree Trail

WHEELER
MEMORIAL

Pond   Trail

Currier Road

Ashumet Farm Trail

Grassy Pond

Grassy Pond Trail

Hooppole Road

FIELD   BARN

FIELD

Ashumet Road

Ashumet Road

N

P

Start/End

0.1 MILE

151   To Mashpee

DESCRIPTION

To enter the sanctuary, follow a dirt-and-gravel road northeast past open fields that in late summer and early fall feature showy displays of goldenrod. After several hundred feet reach a barn and an information board, both on your right. Many barns on the Cape used to house barn swallows, but when these buildings were either torn down or renovated, the swallows lost their homes. This barn has an opening at the top to let these fabulous fliers come and go. To your left are hedges trimmed and decorated to resemble an owl and two lovebirds.

FLORA	FAUNA
This 49-acre sanctuary offers a smorgasbord of botanical delights. Joining the native trees— pitch pine, black oak, white oak, black cherry, red maple, sassafras, tupelo—are 8 species and 65 varieties of holly, more than 1,000 holly trees in all. Shrubs such as arrowwood, highbush blueberry, bayberry, inkberry, wild sarsaparilla, and sweet pepperbush line the route. Other treats include rhododendrons, azaleas, mountain laurel, and nonnative evergreens. Some rare wildflowers, including Plymouth gentian and thread-leaved sundew, an insectivore, grow on the pond's shore.	More than 130 species of birds have been recorded in the sanctuary, including the barn swallows that may greet you near the trailhead. Other winged creatures include butterflies, dragonflies, and damselflies.

Turn right at the barn and pause at the information board, now on your left, to pay the admission fee (for nonmembers) and to peruse the pamphlets for sale, including one with a trail map. Ahead, a sign reading TRAILS directs you to the left. Go straight at the next two junctions, where the Ashumet Farm Trail branches left. Soon descend to the start of the loop the Grassy Pond Trail makes around the pond.

Grassy Pond, like most on the Cape, is a kettle pond. In their undisturbed state, kettle ponds occupy a unique ecological niche as coastal-plain ponds. These freshwater wetlands, which occur along the North Atlantic coast, "are among the most unusual and threatened of Massachusetts natural communities," according to a sanctuary pamphlet. Because a coastal-plain pond's water level is solely dependent on rainfall, Grassy Pond's fluctuating shore is home to specialized plants, including the rare Plymouth gentian and thread-leaved sundew. The pond also provides habitat for rare animals, such as bluet damselflies.

The trail swings left around the pond and soon runs nearly parallel to paved Ashumet and then Hooppole roads. Now pass the first stands of holly, in this case American, for which the sanctuary was named. The various species of hollies collected from around New England that thrive on the sanctuary were planted, beginning in the 1920s, by horticulturist Wilfrid Wheeler, the first Massachusetts commissioner of agriculture. Wheeler owned a 300-acre farm here, and he became known as "the holly man" for his campaign to preserve his favorite trees from habitat loss and holiday-season cutting. After Wheeler died in 1961, a local family purchased the land and donated it to the Massachusetts Audubon Society.

Where the Grassy Pond Trail veers left, bear right on the single-track Mystery Tree Trail and climb gently away from the pond. At a four-way junction with a dirt road, continue straight, now on a wide mowed path. Soon merge with a dirt-and-gravel road joining sharply from the right. Joining the holly trees here is ground-covering ivy, bringing to mind the holiday carol "The Holly and the Ivy": "The holly and the ivy/When they are both full grown/Of all the trees that are in the wood/The holly bears the crown."

After a level stroll, leave the road and turn left onto a trail that passes between two towering holly trees. Next comes a rest bench, left, and then the trail threads its way uphill through a shady, junglelike area full of exotic trees and shrubs. At a four-way junction, where the Mystery Tree Trail goes left, walk straight on the English Holly Trail, a dirt road that descends through a savanna of widely spaced pines, hollies, and rhododendrons. Leave the English Holly Trail by curving left at an upcoming fork and head toward Grassy Pond.

Just before the pond, there is a short trail, right, that leads to a Franklinia tree, a southern import, which blooms beautifully in late summer and early fall. Philadelphia botanists John and William Bartram discovered the species near coastal Georgia and named it for Benjamin Franklin; by 1790 no wild specimens remained. This tree is a descendant of the plants and seeds the Bartrams collected.

When you reach the Grassy Pond Trail, turn right and trace an easy route beside the pond that is lined with stands of highbush blueberry. A rest bench on your left invites a contemplative pause. Stay left at a fork and then, at marker 13, pass a connector on your right that leads to the Ashumet Farm Trail. Close the loop at a T-junction; then turn right and retrace your route uphill to the parking area.

KEY AT-A-GLANCE INFORMATION

GENERAL

DISTANCE 1.6 miles

TYPE OF WALK Loop

DIFFICULTY Easy

TIME TO WALK 1–2 hours

MAPS *Peterson Farm and Beebe Woods,* The 300 Committee; *Woods Hole,* USGS

SCENERY Forest, pond

EXPOSURE TO SUN None

TRAIL TRAFFIC Moderate

TRAIL SURFACE(S) Dirt, wood chips

TRAILS OPEN All year

FEES/PASSES None

FACILITIES None

TRAIL USE

BICYCLES Not allowed

DOGS Allowed on leash

HUNTING Not allowed

HEALTH STATS

NUMBER OF STEPS 3,600

ESTIMATED CALORIES BURNED 171

DIRECTIONS TO TRAILHEAD

From the intersection of Route 28 (North Main Street) and Depot Avenue in Falmouth, go northwest on Depot Avenue, which after 0.1 mile becomes Highfield Drive Go another 0.4 miles to a large paved parking area, which serves the Cape Cod Conservatory and the Highfield Theater. The trailhead is on the northeast corner of the parking area.

Punch Bowl

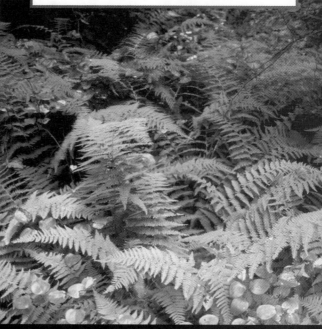

Deep shade and damp soil in Beebe Woods foster fabulous ferns.

WALK SUMMARY

This easy and enjoyable excursion samples a bit of Beebe Woods, making a forested loop to a kettle pond called the Punch Bowl and stopping along the way to study several large boulders, called glacial erratics, left by retreating glaciers. The route also visits the Twin Trees, a remarkable beech with two trunks fused at the base. Plant enthusiasts will enjoy the rich forest environment, which favors a wide variety of native species.

DESCRIPTION

Beebe Woods, nearly 400 acres, was preserved in 1966 thanks to the generosity of Mr. and Mrs. Josiah K. Lilly III, a local couple who are also responsible for the creation, a few years earlier, of the Ashumet

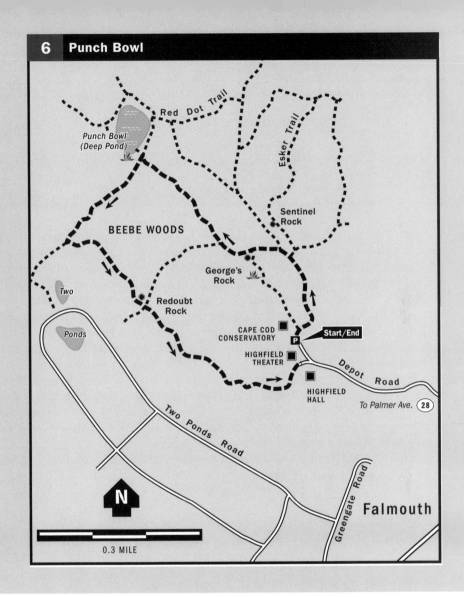

Holly Wildlife Sanctuary. Adjoining Beebe Woods is historic Peterson Farm, which the Town of Falmouth bought in 1998. The purchase was made possible in part by money raised by The 300 Committee, a private nonprofit land trust founded in 1985, exactly 300 years after the incorporation of Falmouth.

Follow a wide dirt trail northeast into the woods, passing a path that joins from the left. The mostly level trail goes through a gap in a stone wall, bends left, and soon comes to the Twin Trees—two tall beeches fused together at the base.

FLORA	FAUNA
The trees here are primarily pitch pine, white pine, black oak, white oak, black cherry, red maple, hickory, sassafras, and American beech. Shrubs include arrowwood, bayberry, black huckleberry, highbush blueberry, sweet pepper-bush, swamp azalea, winterberry, wild raisin, maple-leaved viburnum, and hazelnut. Pond plants include yellow water lilies and pickerel-weed. Spring wildflowers include trailing arbu-tus, or mayflower, and pink lady's slipper.	Mammals found here include gray squirrels, eastern cottontails, chipmunks, foxes, and coyotes.

Just ahead, several trails merge from the right. Continuing the leftward curve, reach a junction with a rest bench and a sign for the Punch Bowl, also called Deep Pond.

Bear left, go through a gap in another stone wall, and soon pass a path, on your left, to George's Rock—a large glacial erratic a few paces left of the trail. Continue straight to a fork and bear right, treading on a cushioning carpet of pine needles. Cresting a rocky rise, descend over eroded, root-crossed ground to a four-way junction beside the Punch Bowl. To visit the pond, go straight. Otherwise, turn left and climb out of the pond's kettle hole on a trail that runs southwest beside a stone wall, right, that marks the boundary of Beebe Woods.

In places unofficial trails diverge from your route: ignore these. Beyond another big glacial boulder is a fork. Bear left and follow a gently rising, winding trail to Redoubt Rock and a four-way junction. Now descend through a beautiful forest, then climb again, passing a path on your right. The trail curves left, threading its way between a stone wall, right, and a rhododendron grove, left. When you reach the Highfield Theater, to your left, veer right and follow a short paved path to Highfield Drive. Turn left and go about 150 feet to the parking area.

Long Pond

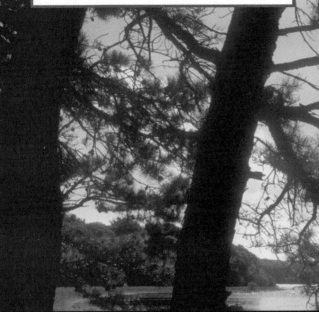

Long Pond, a water-supply area, is in the heart of Falmouth Town Forest.

 KEY AT-A-GLANCE INFORMATION

GENERAL

DISTANCE 3.9 miles

TYPE OF WALK Balloon

DIFFICULTY Moderate

TIME TO WALK 2–3 hours

MAPS *The Moraine Trail Guide*, Cape Cod Pathways; *Falmouth*, USGS

SCENERY Forest, pond

EXPOSURE TO SUN Partial

TRAIL TRAFFIC Light

TRAIL SURFACE(S) Dirt

TRAILS OPEN All year

FEES/PASSES None

FACILITIES Picnic tables, swimming beach; restrooms (seasonal) at the next parking area to the west; children's play area and water on the west side of Goodwill Park

TRAIL USE

BICYCLES Allowed

DOGS Allowed on leash

HUNTING Allowed in season

HEALTH STATS

NUMBER OF STEPS 8,775

ESTIMATED CALORIES BURNED 418

DIRECTIONS TO TRAILHEAD

From the intersection of Main and Gifford streets in Falmouth, take Gifford Street. north 1.2 miles; then turn left into Goodwill Park. Stay left and go 0.3 miles to a large paved parking area, right. The trailhead is on the north side of the park entrance road, just east of the parking area, at an orange metal gate.

WALK SUMMARY

When the Laurentide ice sheet retreated some 15,000 years ago, it left behind in this part of the Cape a wrinkled, rocky landscape dotted with kettle ponds, a landscape very different from the sandy outwash plains found elsewhere on the peninsula. This leg-stretching circuit of Long Pond, which begins in Goodwill Park, takes full advantage of the terrain, dipping close to the pond shore, then rising across hillsides graced with towering trees. Long Pond and the surrounding town forest form the watershed that supplies most of Falmouth's drinking water: access within 100 feet of the pond is prohibited. Note that the Cape Cod Pathways map omits some key trails and junctions and shows some dirt roads as "footpath or trail."

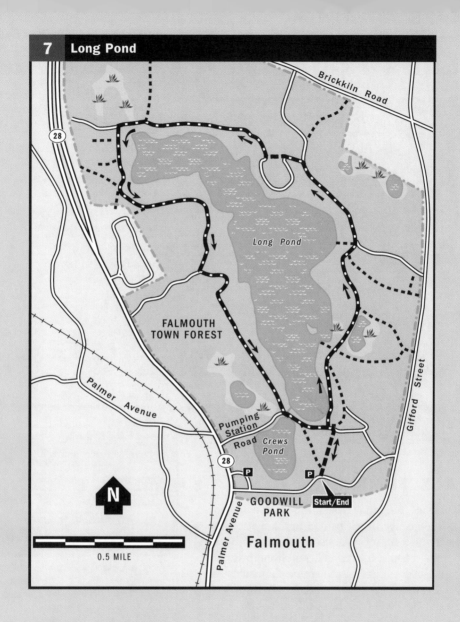

Brickkiln Road

28

Long Pond

FALMOUTH
TOWN FOREST

Palmer Avenue

Pumping
Station

Road Crews
Pond

28

P   P

Gifford Street

N

0.5 MILE

GOODWILL
PARK

Start/End

Palmer Avenue

Falmouth

DESCRIPTION

To begin the walk, go north on a grassy dirt road about 100 feet to junction, where a trail angles left. Continue straight to a T-junction with a dirt road and turn left. After 200 feet or so, turn right onto another dirt road and climb on a gentle grade. Long Pond, on your left, at 150 acres is Falmouth's second largest pond. The pond and its surrounding forest are protected as part of the town's watershed.

Passing a trail to your right, crest a rise and descend. After passing another trail, right, arrive at a four-way junction. Here a dirt road joins on the right and a trail goes left to the pond (stay back 100 feet from the water). Most of Long Pond is fringed with forest right to the water's edge, but in a few places the shoreline is exposed and houses a variety of wildflowers—from common ones, like goldenrods, to rarities such as Plymouth gentian and slender arrowhead.

Continuing a counterclockwise circuit of the pond, soon reach a T-junction with a dirt road. Turn left and follow the road as it curves left, passing a road joining sharply from the right. At about the 1-mile point, arrive at a four-way junction, where a short path leads left to the pond shore, here a sandy beach. Continue straight on the dirt road, gaining elevation as you walk. At the next junction, bear left (west). Just ahead, a dirt road branches left toward the pond, but you stay straight, enjoying a shady, woodland stroll.

Curving right, climb across Falmouth's glacial moraine, part of the Buzzard Bay Moraine, which forms the western edge of Cape Cod. Descend steeply to a junction and merge with a dirt road by angling right. The view, left, extends south across the pond. A rolling course then carries you through a serene realm of tall trees and rocky hillsides, more like the Carolinas than the Cape.

Where a single-track trail joins from the right, your road bends left beside a freshwater marsh. Skirting the northwest corner of Long Pond, climb moderately to a fork and then bear left. Just ahead, the first of two overgrown dirt roads, about 0.15 miles apart, goes right: stay straight at both junctions. At a four-way junction, turn left on a rocky dirt road that rises on a moderate grade. The grade eases after you swing left at a T-junction. Soon pass an overgrown access path on your left that leads to the pond.

Your road passes through a gap in a stone wall, then descends and curves right to a T-junction with another dirt road. Turn left and begin a roller-coaster ride through a forest littered with glacial boulders. Descend to a parking area for several Town of Falmouth facilities and then bear left onto a paved road that runs between Long Pond, left, and Grews Pond, right. Soon close the loop where you began your trek around the pond. Retrace your route to the parking area by going straight, then turning right several hundred feet ahead.

Two-Pond Ramble

Trail offers views of Mashpee Pond, shown here, and Wakeby Pond, its northern neighbor.

WALK SUMMARY

Two large ponds, Mashpee and Wakeby, separated by a peninsula called Conaumet Neck, form the backdrop for this woodsy ramble through a reservation named for its fine stands of American holly. Other trees and shrubs combine to form a botanically rich and diverse environment. Most of the route is well marked with white rectangles affixed to trees beside the trail.

A parking area on South Sandwich Road provides year-round access, but from Memorial Day through Labor Day, 8 a.m. to 5 p.m. (gate is locked promptly without warning), visitors can drive into the heart of the reservation; this shortens the walking distance by about 1.3 miles.

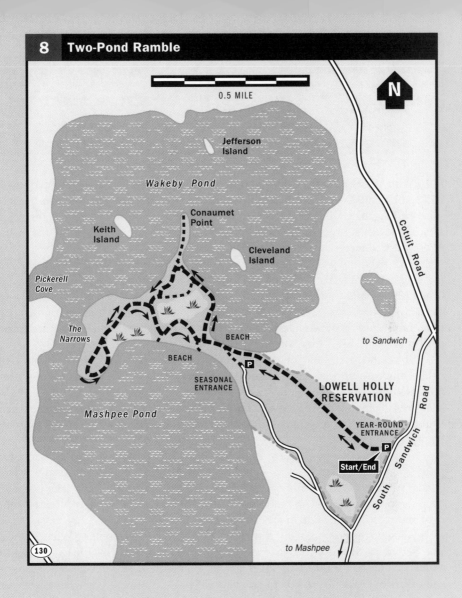

0.5 MILE

N

Jefferson Island

Wakeby Pond

Conaumet Point

Keith Island

Cleveland Island

Pickerell Cove

Cotuit Road

The Narrows

BEACH

to Sandwich

BEACH

SEASONAL ENTRANCE

LOWELL HOLLY RESERVATION

Mashpee Pond

YEAR-ROUND ENTRANCE

South Sandwich Road

Start/End

130

to Mashpee

DESCRIPTION

Pass an information board and follow a well-marked trail into a lush forest containing the reservations namesake trees, American hollies, along with pines, oaks, and other common species. Veer left to cross a ditch, which may be wet, and then meet an unofficial trail joining from the left. Climbing across a hillside that drops right, crest a rise and then descend gently to a junction, where an unofficial trail goes left.

With Wakeby Pond in view, traverse a marshy area, soon arriving at a T-junction beside the pond. Turn left, skirt the shoreline, pass two rest benches, and climb to a seasonal parking area. Find the trail's continuation on the northwest corner of the parking area, where a sign urges caution while swimming, and a tree holds a white trail marker. After your trail merges with a dirt road, the road forks.

Veer right and walk toward Wakeby Pond, with a marshy area to your left. Leave the road by turning right onto a single-track trail, soon reaching a well-situated rest bench with a pond view. Ferns, mushrooms, roots, and leaf litter lend the area a jungle-like feel. A steep, eroded pitch elevates you to a junction with a trail on your left. Continue straight over a ridgetop; then descend to a fork and bear right. Just ahead, at about the 1-mile point, is a T-junction.

To reach the end of Conaumet Point on an overgrown trail with few views, turn right. Otherwise turn left onto a dirt road, soon passing a trail, left. The tree-screened pond is to the right, and a ridge rises left. At the next junction, a fork, bear right and after a few feet join a rough dirt road. On a rolling course, meet the returning end of a short loop on your left. Go straight and descend gently to a clearing, where a view south over Mashpee Pond awaits.

As you face the pond, there is an unofficial trail on the right that goes to a viewpoint overlooking The Narrows—a slim channel separating Mashpee and Wakeby ponds. Wander left (east) through the clearing to find the official trail, here just a faint trace through the trees. The trail curves left and soon closes its short loop. Now bear right and retrace your route to the next junction.

A log on the ground, right, carries an inscription commemorating Wilfrid Wheeler, who served as the first reservation chairman until his death in 1961. Wheeler also planted more than 1,000 holly trees on his Falmouth farm, which later became the Ashumet Holly Wildlife Sanctuary (see page 38).

Continue straight through the junction, now following a level dirt road that curves right. A short trail on the right leads to a lovely beach on the north side of Mashpee Pond. The road bends right and skirts a wet area. Soon another trail joins sharply from the right. Now meet the single-track trail that you explored earlier on your left. From here, continue straight and retrace your route to the parking area.

There is a fee for parking on weekends and holidays. From the intersection of Route 130 and South Sandwich Road in Mashpee, take South Sandwich Road north 0.7 miles; then turn left onto a dirt-and-gravel road. Go 0.2 miles to a fork and bear right. Go another 0.6 miles to a dirt parking area. The trailhead is on the northwest corner of the parking area (see page 48 for details).

West Side Trek

KEY AT-A-GLANCE INFORMATION

GENERAL

DISTANCE 4 miles

TYPE OF WALK Balloon

DIFFICULTY Moderate

TIME TO WALK 2–3 hours

MAPS *Mashpee River Woodlands/South Mashpee Pine Barrens Conservation Area Trail Guide,* Cape Cod Pathways; *Cotuit,* USGS

SCENERY Forest, river

EXPOSURE TO SUN None

TRAIL TRAFFIC Light

TRAIL SURFACE(S) Dirt, sand

TRAILS OPEN All year

FEES/PASSES None

FACILITIES None at the trailhead; picnic table at about 2 miles

TRAIL USE

BICYCLES Allowed

DOGS Allowed on leash

HUNTING Not allowed

HEALTH STATS

NUMBER OF STEPS 9,675

ESTIMATED CALORIES BURNED 461

DIRECTIONS TO TRAILHEAD

From the Route 28 rotary in Mashpee, take Route 28 (signed Route 28 south) northeast for 0.3 miles to Quinaquissett Avenue. Turn right and go 0.1 mile to a parking-area entrance on your right. Continue about 100 feet to a small parking area. The trailhead is on the northwest corner of the parking area, where steps lead downhill. (The trail on the southwest corner of the parking area is the Long River Trail, which explores the east bank of the Mashpee River.)

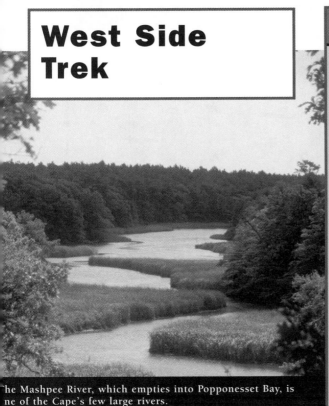

The Mashpee River, which empties into Popponesset Bay, is one of the Cape's few large rivers.

WALK SUMMARY

This sublime walk traces the west bank of the Mashpee River, a scenic waterway linking Mashpee Pond with Popponesset Bay. Several agencies—The Trustees of Reservations, the Town of Mashpee, Massachusetts Division of Fisheries and Wildlife, the Mashpee Wampanoag Tribal Council, Inc., and the Orenda Wildlife Land Trust—have joined together to protect both sides of the river and the adjacent woodlands; trail systems provide public access to each side. The Cape Cod Pathways map includes a trail guide with numbered stops, but there are no numbered markers along the trail. Some of the trails are marked with Cape Cod Pathways signs and are relatively well maintained; others (not used in the walk described below) are nearly impassible because of vegetation.

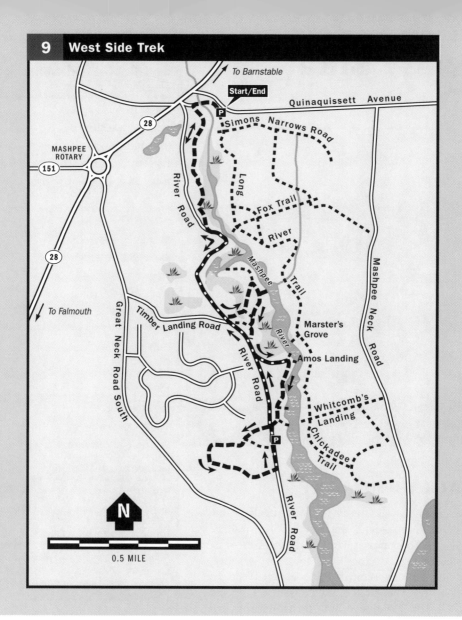

To Barnstable

Start/End

Quinaquissett Avenue

28

Simons Narrows Road

MASHPEE ROTARY

151

Long

Fox Trail

River

River Road

Mashpee

Trail

28

To Falmouth

Timber Landing Road

Great Neck Road South

River Road

Marster's Grove

Amos Landing

Mashpee Neck Road

Whitcomb's Landing

Chickadee Trail

River Road

N

0.5 MILE

DESCRIPTION

To begin, descend through a dense stand of trees and shrubs to a power-line access road and then cross a wet area via a wooden bridge. Ahead the trail curves left and joins a dirt road, which soon crosses a bridge over the Mashpee River. Prior to the 20th century, this was a main thoroughfare across the river. Where a sign welcomes you to the Mashpee River Reservation, turn left on a faint trail that stays just right of the sign.

In a clearing, merge with a loop at the end of a dirt road. Two trails depart from the end of the loop—a short one going to the river, left, and your route, which goes straight. Check the tall pines nearby; some are riddled with woodpecker holes. Follow the trail through a narrow corridor of shrubs, soon crossing the outlet stream from Trout Pond and several wet areas via a series of short bridges. The pond once was used as a fish hatchery by the former owners of the riverfront property—the Mashpee River Trout Club and Boston lawyer John Farley.

Passing an unofficial trail on your right, gain elevation on a moderate grade, soon reaching a rest bench that commands a superb view of the Mashpee River, which flows southward a few miles to Popponesset Bay. In addition to several species of trout and warm-water fish, the river has a run of alewives, which are anadromous fish that migrate in spring from salt water to spawn in freshwater ponds. Ahead, another unofficial trail goes right, but you'll stay straight and follow a rolling course. At a junction with River Road, bear left. The dirt road swings right to skirt Canaway Cove, which marks tidewater's farthest inland reach.

After crossing a culvert, pass a road on your left that is not shown on the map. Old cranberry bogs, once irrigated with river water, are on your right. At about the 1-mile point, where dirt Timber Landing Road joins sharply from the right, continue straight. After about 75 feet, arrive at a four-way junction. Turn hard left on a dirt road, go about 200 feet, and then turn right onto a single-track trail. Climb past a rest bench on your right and then turn sharply left at a junction.

Now descend on a single-track trail to a T-junction and turn right. Several hundred feet ahead, an overgrown path to the river splits left, but you'll go straight. Stay on track as paths diverge—first left, then right—and enjoy a rolling stroll to the next T-junction (shown incorrectly on the Cape Cod Pathways map as going straight and the overgrown dirt road joining from the right) with an overgrown dirt road. Bear left, go a few hundred feet to the road's end, and then follow a trail that curves right and descends to River Road.

Here turn left onto River Road, descend to cross a culvert, and then pass a path on your right that leads to a paved road. Just ahead, meet a road to Amos Landing at a fork. Angle left and soon cross another culvert. Just before the landing, a trail departs right; you will use this in a few minutes. For now, continue straight to a fork; views of the river and the adjacent salt marsh are available at the end of each of the fork's branches (a rest bench rewards lefties). Now retrace your route to the trail mentioned earlier in this paragraph.

Go left onto the trail, pass a rest bench with a fine river view, and then snake your way steeply uphill to a picnic table. Beyond the table a path forks left, but you'll angle right and soon reach level ground near a rest bench. The trail splits to pass around a tall pitch pine, then arrives at a four-way junction with River Road. An interpretive panel here explains the importance of estuaries, where freshwater and saltwater meet.

Cross the road and find the trail's continuation in a forest presided over by stately white pines. The trail curves left, descends, then climbs past a connector to Holland Mill Road in the South Mashpee Pine Barrens (see page 58). Soon, at about the 2.4-mile point you'll reach River Road, here paved. Turn left and retrace your route to the four-way junction with the interpretive panel mentioned in the above paragraph.

Stay on River Road, remembering to stay right at the fork with Timber Landing Road (just past an Orenda Land Trust sign, left). Now retrace your route around Canaway Cove to the junction where you first joined River Road (a housing development is visible on the left here). Turn right on the single-track trail and retrace your route to the parking area.

Great Flat Pond Trail

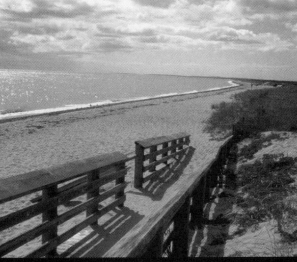

...th Cape Beach State Park offers walking trails and ...ess to Vineyard Sound.

WALK SUMMARY

This short but botanically rich walk beckons beach-goers who may want a brief break from a day spent enjoying the sun and sand beside Vineyard Sound. The state park is part of the Falmouth-based Waquoit Bay National Estuarine Research and Reserve, which, according to its Web site, "provides long-term pro-tection to the habitat and resources of this represen-tative estuarine ecosystem." The trails here, some overgrown (long pants advised), are reserved for walking only. Guided walks are offered during the summer. The State Park and the nearby Town of Mashpee beach provide access to Vineyard Sound.

KEY AT-A-GLANCE INFORMATION

GENERAL

DISTANCE 1.3 miles

TYPE OF WALK Balloon

DIFFICULTY Easy

TIME TO WALK 1 hour or less

MAPS *South Cape Beach,* from Mashpee Planning Department; *Falmouth,* USGS

SCENERY Forest, salt marsh, scrub woodland

EXPOSURE TO SUN Partial

TRAIL TRAFFIC Light

TRAIL SURFACE(S) Dirt

TRAILS OPEN All year; parking closed Columbus Day–Patriots Day (mid-April)

FEES/PASSES Parking fee (seasonal)

FACILITIES Toilets (seasonal); wheel-chair access to beach during summer

TRAIL USE

BICYCLES Trails not suitable for bicycles

DOGS Allowed on leash

HUNTING Allowed in season

HEALTH STATS

NUMBER OF STEPS 2,925

ESTIMATED CALORIES BURNED 139

DIRECTIONS TO TRAILHEAD

From the Route 28 rotary in Mashpee, take Great Neck Road south, signed for New Seabury. Go 2.7 miles to an intersection, right, with Red Brook Road. Veer slightly left, now on Great Oak Road. Go 2.1 miles and turn left into the State Park. Go 0.2 miles to an intersection and turn left (the road going straight goes to a Mashpee town beach). Go 0.4 miles to the state-park parking area. The trailhead is on the right (east) side of the entrance road, about 100 yards north of parking area.

Note: When the state-park parking area is closed, parking is available at the town beach; no parking sticker required then.

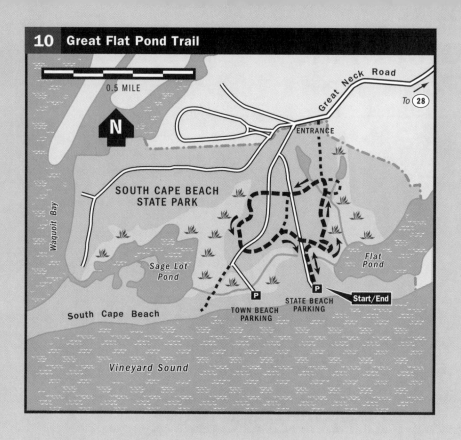

SOUTH CAPE BEACH
STATE PARK

Waquoit Bay

ENTRANCE

Great Neck Road

To (28)

0.5 MILE

N

Sage Lot
Pond

Flat
Pond

P

P

Start/End

TOWN BEACH
PARKING

STATE BEACH
PARKING

South Cape Beach

Vineyard Sound

DESCRIPTION

From the trailhead, begin by following a trail east into a pitch pine–scrub oak woodland, reach a T-junction, and turn right. The curvy trail meanders on a level course beside the marsh bordering Flat Pond. After a boardwalk helps you across a wet area, thread your way through a tunnel of shrubs. Where a faint trace goes straight, a trail marker directs you left.

The trail flirts with the marsh for a while, then returns to the woodland. When you reach the paved state-park entrance road, cross it and continue on a level trail into the pines. After a few hundred feet, cross another paved road—it goes to the town beach—and take a trail into a scrub woodland, where the trees' shorter stature testifies to the power of coastal storms.

Soon you'll reach a town parking area, signed BAYBERRY. Stay right and walk to the parking area's south end. Go about 25 feet to the paved road, cross it, and find the trail's continuation. With a large salt marsh on the right, traverse a brushy corridor, cross a short bridge over a creek, and then stroll through a

Pitch pine, black oak, sassafras, red maple, and tupelo dominate the woodlands. Shrubs include high-bush blueberry, inkberry, black huckleberry, bayberry, wild raisin, checkerberry, sweet pepperbush, sheep laurel, swamp azalea, scrub oak, dwarf chestnut oak, and chokeberry. Poison ivy, greenbrier, and Virginia creeper twine beside the trail.

possibly wet area, where boards have been placed over the trail (step carefully: some of the boards are unanchored).

At a T-junction, signed either way, turn right and reenter dense woodland. Cross the state-park entrance road and continue on a trail; then close the loop and turn sharply right to retrace your route to the trailhead.

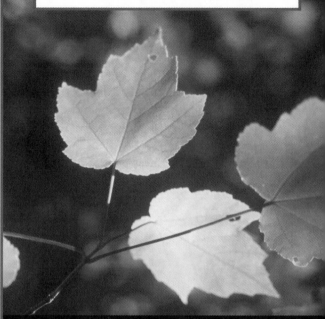

Red maple is a common Cape tree with a wide distribution the East Coast, found from Maine to Florida.

KEY AT-A-GLANCE INFORMATION

GENERAL

DISTANCE 3.7 miles

TYPE OF WALK Balloon

DIFFICULTY Moderate

TIME TO WALK 2–3 hours

MAPS *Mashpee River Woodlands/South Mashpee Pine Barrens Conservation Area Trail Guide,* Cape Cod Pathways; *Cotuit,* USGS

SCENERY Freshwater marsh, pine barrens

EXPOSURE TO SUN Partial

TRAIL TRAFFIC Light; some vehicles

TRAIL SURFACE(S) Dirt, sand

TRAILS OPEN All year

FEES/PASSES None

FACILITIES None

TRAIL USE

BICYCLES Allowed

DOGS Allowed on leash

HUNTING Not allowed

HEALTH STATS

NUMBER OF STEPS 8,325

ESTIMATED CALORIES BURNED 396

DIRECTIONS TO TRAILHEAD

From the Route 28 rotary in Mashpee, take Great Neck Road south, signed for New Seabury. Go 1.8 miles to Holland Mill Road, an unsigned dirt road, right. Go several hundred feet and park beside the road on the left. Do not park in the adjacent Wampanoag Tribal Council parking area. The route follows Holland Mill Road to the west.

Pine Barrens

WALK SUMMARY

The South Mashpee Pine Barrens Conservation Area is an island of open space amid rapid and extensive residential development. The dirt roads and trails through this special area, which is part of the Mashpee National Wildlife Refuge, take visitors through a landscape that is anything but "barren." A diversity of habitats, including rare Atlantic white-cedar swamps, provides a variety of plants and animals to study and enjoy. This walk is best done on a cool day.

Note: Part of the route traverses lands of the Wampanoag Tribal Council, which has granted public access. Please stay on the road and do not enter or disturb tribal areas or structures.

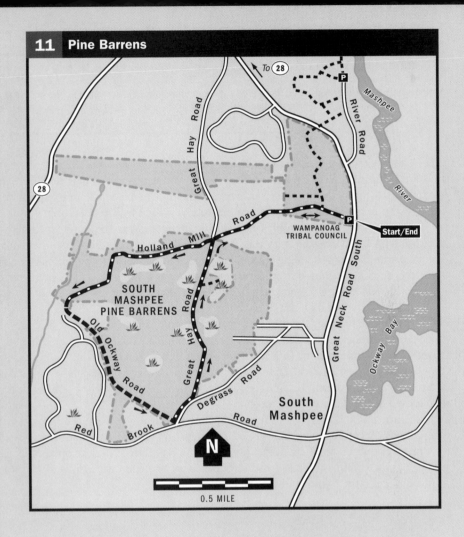

To 28

River Road

Mashpee

River

Great Hay Road

28

Road

Holland Mill

WAMPANOAG
TRIBAL COUNCIL

P

Start/End

SOUTH
MASHPEE
PINE BARRENS

Great Hay Road

Great Neck Road South

Ockway Bay

Old Ockway Road

Degrass Road

South
Mashpee

Red Brook

Road

N

0.5 MILE

DESCRIPTION

Follow the level dirt road, which soon curves left and descends past a trail on your right that connects to the Mashpee River Woodlands trail system. Soon pass a Wampanoag ceremonial area on your left. The Wampanoags—the name means "People of the First Light"—and their ancestors have lived in this area for at least 10,000 years. It was the Wampanoag who helped the Pilgrims survive after they landed in Provincetown in 1620 and later settled in Plymouth. Please stay on the road and do not enter the site.

FLORA

In addition to the pitch pine and scrub oak that predominate in the pine barrens, the route also passes stands of black oak, white oak, black cherry, red maple, and sassafras. Shrubs include bearberry, black huckleberry, bayberry, sheep laurel, dwarf sumac, dwarf chestnut oak, wild sarsaparilla, sweet fern, and chokeberry. Goldenrods and asters add color in late summer and fall.

Unlike the more densely forested areas on the Upper Cape, the Mashpee Pine Barrens are reminiscent of the pitch pine–scrub oak woodlands of Wellfleet and Truro. But as in those towns, oaks and other hardwoods proliferate here and will one day dominate the forest, unless this process, called succession, is altered by fire or cutting.

At a four-way junction with Great Hay Road, go straight and begin to climb on a narrowing track. An excavation on your right is used as a trash dump—not a particularly scenic feature. Now on a rolling course, pass a trail that cuts sharply right. Stay left at a fork; the branches rejoin after 100 yards or so. With a housing development on the right, swing left, passing a gate and a fire hydrant. After another fire hydrant and a gate, your trail curves left and another trail departs right.

Just before reaching a paved turn-around in a housing development, bear left on a trail, shown on the map as Old Ockway Road, through a wooded area. The trail ends at paved Degrass Road, near its intersection with Red Brook Road. Turn left and walk along the shoulder of Degrass Road, facing oncoming traffic. When you reach Great Hay Road, a dirt road, angle left (and be alert for vehicles). Areas beside this road, too, suffer from being used as unofficial trash dumps.

Gentle ups and downs keep the walking interesting as you head north past a series of wetlands. According to the Cape Cod Pathways trail guide, five Atlantic white-cedar swamps, relatively rare on the Cape, border Great Hay Road. No developed trails exist through these swamps. When you reach the four-way junction with Holland Mill Road, turn right and retrace your route to the parking area.

Cape Cod:
Mid-Cape

GENERAL

DISTANCE 2 miles

TYPE OF WALK Balloon

DIFFICULTY Easy

TIME TO WALK 1–2 hours

MAPS "Bridge Creek Conservation Area" in *A Hiker's Guide to Town of Barnstable Conservation Lands and Sandy Neck*, Barnstable Conservation Commission, or print from town Web site; *Hyannis*, USGS

SCENERY Forest

EXPOSURE TO SUN Partial

TRAIL TRAFFIC Light

TRAIL SURFACE(S) Dirt

TRAILS OPEN All year

FEES/PASSES None

FACILITIES None

TRAIL USE

BICYCLES Allowed; some trails may be closed to bicycles during wet weather

DOGS Allowed on leash or under voice control

HUNTING Allowed in season in the conservation area but not in the wildlife sanctuary

HEALTH STATS

NUMBER OF STEPS 4,500

ESTIMATED CALORIES BURNED 214

DIRECTIONS TO TRAILHEAD

From Route 6 in West Barnstable, take Exit 5 and follow Route 149 north 0.1 mile to Church Street. Turn right, go 0.3 miles, bear slightly left to stay on Church Street, and go another 0.4 miles to a small gravel parking area, left. The trailhead is on the east side of the parking area.

East Side Ramble

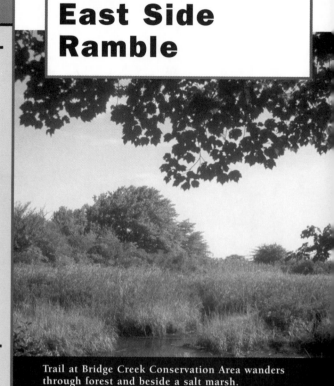

Trail at Bridge Creek Conservation Area wanders through forest and beside a salt marsh.

WALK SUMMARY

Bordering the tiny Jenkins Wildlife Sanctuary, this ample conservation area is a treasure trove of native trees, shrubs, and wildflowers. The walk described below traverses the east side of the area through forest and beside marshes; another trail leaves from the west side of the parking area and goes to a parking area next to the West Barnstable Fire Station on Route 149.

DESCRIPTION

From the parking area, follow a wide dirt trail that soon curves left (northeast), away from Church Street, and descends gently into a beautiful forest. At a junction, angle right and enjoy a level walk beside an old stone wall and the headwaters of Bridge Creek. Continue straight at the next junction

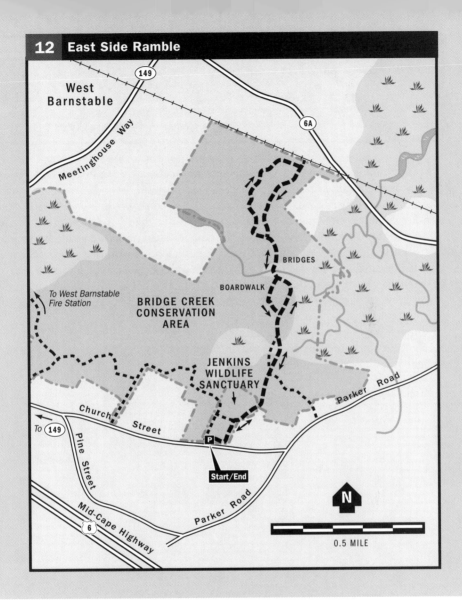

West
Barnstable

149

6A

To West Barnstable
Fire Station

BRIDGES

BOARDWALK

BRIDGE CREEK
CONSERVATION
AREA

JENKINS
WILDLIFE
SANCTUARY

Parker Road

Church Street

To 149

Pine Street

P

Start/End

Mid-Cape Highway

6

Parker Road

N

0.5 MILE

and cross a possibly wet area on wooden planks. Where a trail from Parker Road joins on the right, stay straight and navigate a tunnel of trees and shrubs.

Curve left to a junction, turn right, and use a short boardwalk to cross a swampy area. Pass through a gap in a stone wall and then meet the trail from the previous junction joining on your left. Descend to another possibly wet area—wooden planks will help you across. A rest bench offers a view of an adjacent marsh, which has stands of common reeds and cattails. Poison sumac grows nearby, so stay on the trail.

Turn right at the next junction; then cross a wet area via two boardwalks. Between the boardwalks, another rest bench provides a marsh view. Beyond them, climb a curvy course through dense forest. Now you pass a trail departing right; you will return on it in a few minutes. Go through a gap in a stone wall; then bend right and traverse a shrubby area full of poison ivy—stay on the trail. Railroad tracks are nearby, to your left.

At a T-junction, turn right. In a sandy clearing dotted with trees, follow the indistinct trail by angling right. Descend past a stone wall; then close the loop and turn left. Now retrace your route to the junction just past the two boardwalks. Turn right and use a boardwalk to traverse a red maple swamp, where tupelos join to add a splash of color in fall. Continue straight, passing an unofficial trail going right. Now descend, curve left, go through a gap in a stone wall, and rejoin the trail you were on earlier. From here, retrace your route to the parking area, remembering to stay left at the first fork and straight at the next three junctions.

Forest Foray

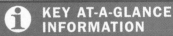
KEY AT-A-GLANCE INFORMATION

GENERAL

DISTANCE 2.2 miles

TYPE OF WALK Balloon

DIFFICULTY Moderate

TIME TO WALK 1–2 hours

MAPS "Old Jail Lane Conservation Area" in *A Hiker's Guide to Town of Barnstable Conservation Lands and Sandy Neck*, Barnstable Conservation Commission, or print from town Web site; *Hyannis*, USGS

SCENERY Forest

EXPOSURE TO SUN None

TRAIL TRAFFIC Light

TRAIL SURFACE(S) Dirt

TRAILS OPEN All year

FEES/PASSES None

FACILITIES None

TRAIL USE

BICYCLES Allowed

DOGS Allowed on leash or under voice control

HUNTING Allowed in season

HEALTH STATS

NUMBER OF STEPS 4,950

ESTIMATED CALORIES BURNED 236

DIRECTIONS TO TRAILHEAD

From Route 6 in Barnstable, take Exit 6 and follow Route 132 southeast 1.4 miles to Phinney's Lane. Turn left, go 1 mile (just after passing under Route 6), and turn left on Old Jail Lane. Go 0.5 miles and turn left on a dirt road leading to a small dirt parking area, right.

From the intersection (hard to see) of Route 6A and Old Jail Lane in Barnstable, take Old Jail Lane south 0.6 miles; then turn right on a dirt road leading to a small dirt parking area, right. The trailhead is on the southwest side of the parking area.

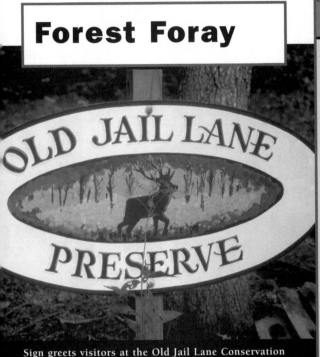

Sign greets visitors at the Old Jail Lane Conservation area, which is near the busy village of Hyannis.

WALK SUMMARY

This exploration of a densely wooded conservation area tucked between Route 6 and Route 6A shows the value of protecting parcels of open space amid busy residential and commercial zones. Ramble along old dirt roads beside stands of tall pines and oaks, with only birdsong for a soundtrack, and the hustle and bustle of the Cape's biggest town, Barnstable, and its busiest village, Hyannis, all but disappear.

DESCRIPTION

Follow the dirt road southwest from the parking area, past a few homes, and after a few hundred feet reach a metal gate. Go left around it and follow a trail that skirts a grassy meadow. Now regain the dirt road, which is bordered by rocks and boulders, evidence of the glacial moraine that formed this part of the Cape.

65

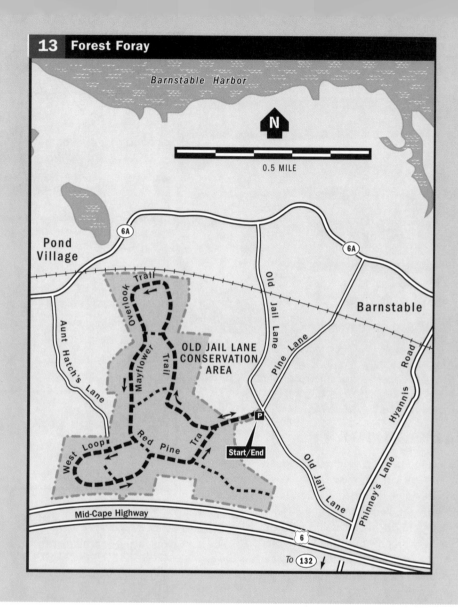

At a fork there is a rough sketch map of the area, showing trail names. Bear right on the Red Pine Trail, an overgrown dirt road, and follow a rolling course through dense forest. The road curves right to an unsigned junction, where the Red Pine Trail goes left. Continue straight, now on the Mayflower Trail. Climb moderately, then drop to a low spot. Just beyond is a fork. Here the Mayflower Trail goes left, but you veer right on the Overlook Trail. (To shorten the walk by about 0.4 miles, turn left on the Mayflower Trail and follow the route description below.)

<table>
<tr><td>

FLORA

Pitch pine, black oak, white oak, black cherry, shadbush, sassafras, bigtooth aspen, American holly, and autumn olive are among the trees thriving here. Shrubs include highbush blueberry, black huckleberry, arrowwood, bayberry, chokeberry, and dwarf sumac. Poison ivy, greenbrier, Virginia creeper, and wild grape lurk just off, and sometimes on, the trail.

</td><td>

FAUNA

Blue jays, black-capped chickadees, and gray catbirds call this area home. Listen for the "keeer" cry of a red-tailed hawk overhead. Birdhouses here and there encourage cavity nesters.

</td></tr>
</table>

A roller-coaster ride over rough ground puts you atop a hill where, despite the trail name, the views are mostly of the surrounding forest. Descend to a junction and rejoin the Mayflower Trail by going straight. Pass the Red Pine Trail on your left and soon meet the West Loop, on your right, and a more detailed trailside map. (To shorten the walk by about 0.5 miles, stay straight on the Red Pine Trail and follow the route description below.)

Turn right onto the West Loop. A hilly ramble takes you past Aunt Hatch's Lane, around a leftward bend, and to a T-junction with the Red Pine Trail. Here turn right, continue through forest to the next junction, and then angle sharply left to stay on the Red Pine Trail. Climb gently, close the loop, and then bear right and retrace your route to the parking area.

GENERAL

DISTANCE 11.2 miles

TYPE OF WALK Balloon

DIFFICULTY Difficult

TIME TO WALK 5–6 hours

MAPS "Sandy Neck" in *A Hiker's Guide to Town of Barnstable Conservation Lands and Sandy Neck*, Barnstable Conservation Commission, or print from town Web site; *Sandwich* and *Hyannis*, USGS

SCENERY Barrier beach, dunes, Cape Cod Bay, forest, salt marsh

EXPOSURE TO SUN Full

TRAIL TRAFFIC Light

TRAIL SURFACE(S) Dirt, sand

TRAILS OPEN All year

FEES/PASSES None

FACILITIES None at trailhead; toilets at beach parking area

TRAIL USE

BICYCLES Allowed but not advised because of soft sand

DOGS On leash March 1–September 15; leashed or under direct voice control at all other times; not allowed on swimming beach or in beach parking area

HUNTING Allowed in season

HEALTH STATS

NUMBER OF STEPS 25,200

ESTIMATED CALORIES BURNED 1,200

DIRECTIONS TO TRAILHEAD

From Route 6 in West Barnstable, take Exit 5 and follow Route 149 north 1 mile to Route 6A. Turn left, go 2 miles (after entering Sandwich), and turn right on Sandy Neck Road. At 0.8 miles, you reach the Sandy Neck ranger station. There are 3 parking spaces for trail users, just west of the ranger station; parking here is free. If these are full, there are 2 large parking areas at the beach, 0.3 miles ahead. Parking here is free for Barnstable residents; there is a fee in summer for nonresidents.

Great Marshes to Cape Cod Bay

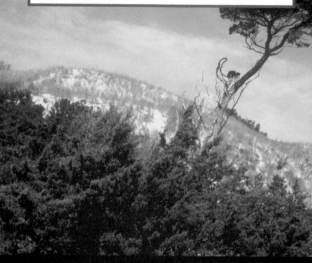

Lone eastern red cedar rises above sand dunes bordering the Marsh Trail.

WALK SUMMARY

This classic Cape walk, best done on a cool day, explores a pristine 6-mile peninsula, actually a barrier beach, that juts eastward from the Sandwich/Barnstable line and forms the sheltering northern border of the Great Marshes and then of Barnstable Harbor. Your route, on dirt roads called "trails," traces the marsh side first, then crosses the peninsula and returns via the shore of Cape Cod Bay.

DESCRIPTION

The trailhead is just southeast of the ranger station, just across Sandy Neck Road, at a gated dirt road. A mileage sign and an information board are beside the trailhead. Head east on the Marsh Trail, a dirt road patched in places with small rocks. The road borders the Great Marshes, 8,000 acres of salt

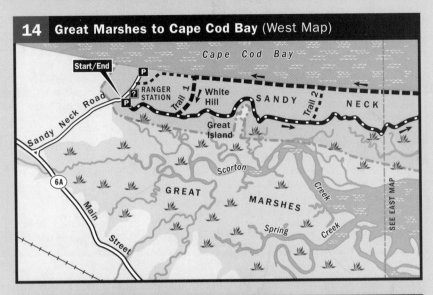

14 **Great Marshes to Cape Cod Bay** (West Map)

Cape Cod Bay

Start/End

RANGER STATION

White Hill

Trail 1

Great Island

S A N D Y   N E C K

Trail 2

Sandy Neck Road

6A

Main

Street

Scorton

G R E A T   M A R S H E S   Creek

Spring   Creek

SEE EAST MAP

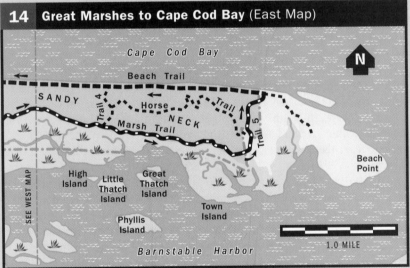

14 **Great Marshes to Cape Cod Bay** (East Map)

N

Cape Cod Bay

Beach Trail

S A N D Y

Trail 4

Horse

Marsh Trail

N E C K

Trail

Trail 5

Beach Point

SEE WEST MAP

High Island   Little Thatch Island   Great Thatch Island

Town Island

Phyllis Island

Barnstable Harbor

1.0 MILE

marsh cut by miles of sinuous tidal creeks and channels—a vast wildlife habitat that shelters ducks, geese, herons, egrets, and shorebirds and provides a hunting ground for raptors such as hawks and falcons. To your left are rolling dunes, built up over eons by tons upon tons of wind-deposited sand. Beyond them, to the north, lies Cape Cod Bay.

Where the road forks, take either branch, unless the lower branch is flooded. The circular, grass-free bodies of water in the marsh are called salt

FLORA	FAUNA
This walk explores a variety of habitats, including forest, dune, salt marsh, and seashore, and flora that is equally varied. Forest species include pitch pine, scrub oak, black oak, white oak, eastern red cedar, black cherry, autumn olive, shadbush, sassafras, and black huckleberry. Growing in or near the dunes and seashore are bayberry, beach plum, dwarf sumac, poison ivy, poverty grass, greenbrier, Virginia creeper, dusty miller, seabeach sandwort, seaside spurge, sea rocket, American beach grass, and goldenrod. In the salt marsh, look for saltwater cordgrass, salt hay, spike grass, marsh lavender, marsh elder, salt-marsh aster, glasswort, and sea blite.	Many water birds, waders, and shorebirds frequent the Great Marshes and the shore of Cape Cod Bay, but Sandy Neck has other habitats—forests, thickets, dunes—that attract songbirds. Some of these are blue jays, red-winged blackbirds, crows, Northern flickers, gray catbirds, dark-eyed juncos, horned larks, warblers, finches, and sparrows. Raptors, including osprey, northern harriers, and Cooper's hawks, may appear just about anywhere.

pannes; they are the result of high salinity from evaporation killing marsh grasses and exposing the underlying peat. After about 0.5 miles, you'll pass Trail 1, left. At the next junction, a fork, stay left. Where the road climbs slightly, a fine view unfolds across the marsh to the highlands of Sandwich and Barnstable, the glacial-moraine backbone of the Cape.

The road winds past the first of a handful of cabins, along with a few hunting shacks, scattered along the marsh. At about 2 miles, pass Trail 2, which angles left. The deeper creeks in the marsh are bordered by saltwater cordgrass, which is more salt tolerant than its cousin, salt hay, found in the marsh's higher elevations. Soon you'll come to a cabin with a splendid assortment of birdhouses nearby, perhaps for mosquito control. In places, there are patches of salt marsh to the left of the road, drained and filled via culverts.

At about 3.5 miles, cross a concrete bridge over a creek; then stroll another 0.5 miles to Trail 4, which goes left. Continuing straight, pass extensive dunes, left, carpeted with poison ivy, bayberry, and poverty grass. The island-dotted upper reaches of Barnstable Harbor are to your right. An osprey pole, perhaps with a nest on top, rises from the marsh. The return of these magnificent fish-eating hawks from the brink of extinction induced by DDT is an environmental triumph, and nesting poles in the Cape's marshes played an important role.

A stand of pitch pines offers the route's first shade, and soon you curve left and reach a junction at the end of the Marsh Trail. Here, at about 5.5 miles, you'll join Trail 5 by going straight; there is also a dirt road going right that skirts the edge of the marsh. Your route, mostly on soft sand, now swings north and cuts across the widest part of Sandy Neck. The stunted pitch pines here have large circular skirts of branches that extend outward at ground level, perhaps as a defense against sandblasting, or perhaps to better anchor themselves in the wind.

After a dirt road joins sharply from the right, your route makes several big S-bends and arrives at a four-way junction. An equestrian trail is left, and a dirt road goes right, but you continue straight. A small wild cranberry bog is to the right of the road, in a low-lying area. After passing another dirt road, to your right, your road curves right and enters a shady corridor of pines. Now emerging into a more open habitat, climb to a junction at about 6 miles.

Angle left on a sandy road, traverse a stretch of dunes, and descend to the scenic shore of Cape Cod Bay. Turn left and follow a four-wheel-drive track, which is separated from the dunes by a line of posts and rope. The gently sloping beach leads to the water's edge—or mudflats and sandbars if the tide is low—where you may spot gulls, terns, or shorebirds. On a clear day, binoculars will help you pick out Provincetown's Pilgrim Monument, slightly east of north and more than 20 miles away.

At about 7.5 miles, pass Trail 4 on your left. The Cape Cod Canal, marked by a power-station tower and the Sagamore Bridge, is a bit north of west, about 9 miles away. Where Trail 2 goes left, at just past 9 miles, you continue straight. A little more than a mile ahead, turn left on Trail 1 and negotiate the hilly dunes via a soft-sand road and, where the road all but disappears, by following footprints. When you reach the Marsh Trail, turn right and retrace your route to the parking area.

KEY AT-A-GLANCE INFORMATION

GENERAL

DISTANCE 3.9 miles

TYPE OF WALK Balloon

DIFFICULTY Moderate

TIME TO WALK 2–3 hours

MAPS "West Barnstable Conservation Area" in *A Hiker's Guide to Town of Barnstable Conservation Lands and Sandy Neck*, Barnstable Conservation Commission, or print from town Web site; *Sandwich*, USGS

SCENERY Forest

EXPOSURE TO SUN None

TRAIL TRAFFIC Light

TRAIL SURFACE(S) Dirt

TRAILS OPEN All year

FEES/PASSES None

FACILITIES None

TRAIL USE

BICYCLES Allowed

DOGS Allowed on leash or under voice control

HUNTING Allowed in season

HEALTH STATS

NUMBER OF STEPS 8,775

ESTIMATED CALORIES BURNED 418

DIRECTIONS TO TRAILHEAD

From Route 6 in West Barnstable, take Exit 5, follow Route 149 south 0.3 miles to a fork, and bear right. Go another 0.5 miles to Popple Bottom Road, turn sharply right, and go about 100 feet to a small gravel parking area, right, with space for about 3 cars (have another destination planned if this parking area is full). The trailhead is on the north side of the parking area, at a gap in a split-rail fence.

Moraine Trek

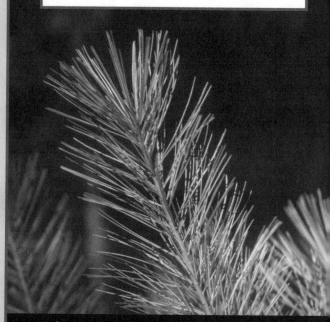

Pitch pines are well represented in Cape forests, often gro in association with various oaks.

WALK SUMMARY

This is one of the few walks in this book that may actually deserve the name "hike," both because of the rolling nature of the terrain and the steepness of individual sections of trail. So a spirit of adventure is in order, along with sturdy boots. Visitors are rewarded with a trek through a magnificent pine-and-hardwood forest, which may whet the appetite for further explorations of this 1,114-acre conservation area crisscrossed by many miles of trails.

DESCRIPTION

Follow a narrow dirt trail that meanders through the woods and curves left to meet Popple Bottom Road, here dirt. Turn right and soon reach a four-way junction, where a dirt road angles right and a trail goes left. Continue walking straight to the next

15 Moraine Trek

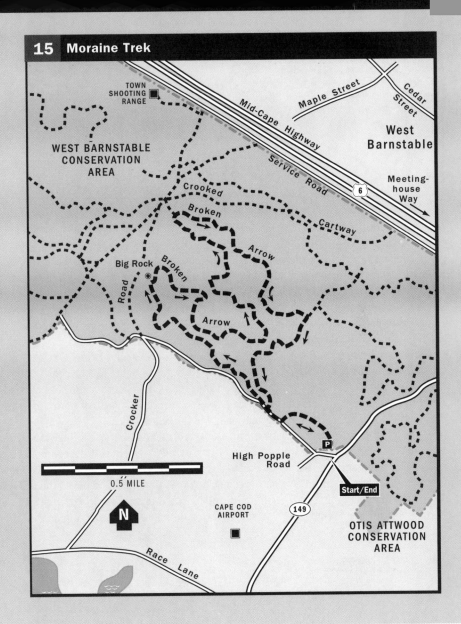

TOWN SHOOTING RANGE

WEST BARNSTABLE CONSERVATION AREA

Mid-Cape Highway

Maple Street

Cedar Street

Service Road

West Barnstable

6

Meeting-house Way

Crooked

Broken

Cartway

Arrow

Big Rock

Broken

Road

Arrow

Arrow

Crocker

High Popple Road

P

0.5 MILE

N

CAPE COD AIRPORT

149

Start/End

Race Lane

OTIS ATTWOOD CONSERVATION AREA

junction, also a four-way, where you turn right on a single-track trail, formerly called the Trail of Tears but now shown on the Web site map as Broken Arrow.

Carpeted with pine needles, the trail roller-coasters across a landscape sculpted by the Laurentide ice sheet—nearby Route 6 follows the top of a gla-cial moraine that runs generally east–west along the length of the Cape from Sandwich about half way to the Atlantic Ocean. Rocks and boulders beside the

FLORA	FAUNA
Dense forest characterizes this conservation area, with trees such as pitch pine, white pine, black oak, white oak, black cherry, eastern red cedar, red maple, hickory, gray birch, speckled alder, American holly, and sassafras. Shrubs here include arrowwood, bayberry, black huckleberry, sheep laurel, and highbush blueberry.	Dead trees, or snags, provide homes for cavity nesters, including black-capped chickadees and woodpeckers. Other common birds here include blue jays, northern flickers, and northern cardinals. Look carefully on the forest floor and you may spot the nest of an eastern woodrat, or packrat—a circular mound of debris, three to four feet in diameter and six to eight inches high, with an entrance hole.

trail were deposited here by the ice sheet's snout as it pushed southward, stopped, and then retreated.

Bear right at a fork; the branches soon rejoin. At about 1 mile, pass a trail going right (not shown on the map) and soon reach a junction beside a large boulder on the left, whose summit affords views of the surrounding forest but not much else. Continue straight, keeping the rock on your left; then curve right and climb steeply. The trail is now within earshot of busy Route 6 and also a Town of Barnstable shooting range, so don't be alarmed if you hear gunfire (unless it is hunting season).

The trail twists, turns, dips, and climbs. Walking east just below a ridgetop, you curve left to a junction and then pass a faint path going right. Just beyond, your trail curves left almost 180 degrees, traverses a valley, and climbs across the side of a ridge. Bending right, the trail exits the valley via a steep climb slightly west of north. After more elevations, declinations, and peregrinations, you'll reach a fork.

Bear right and descend eastward into a ravine, meeting a trail joining sharply from the left. A rolling course soon puts you atop a rocky ridge, which you descend on a steep grade. More ups and downs, followed by several hairpin turns, bring you to a four-way junction (shown as a T-junction on the map), just past the 3-mile point, with a dirt road. Turn right and, passing a trail going right, follow the dirt road about 0.4 miles to meet Popple Bottom Road. Here turn left and retrace your route to the parking area.

Grand Traverse

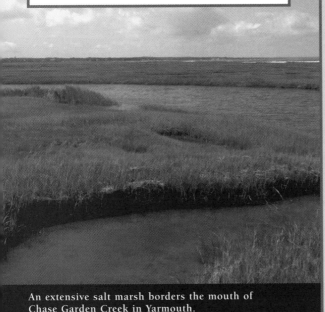

An extensive salt marsh borders the mouth of Chase Garden Creek in Yarmouth.

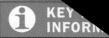

KEY INFORMATION

GENERAL

DISTANCE 3.2 miles

TYPE OF WALK Balloon

DIFFICULTY Moderate

TIME TO WALK 1–2 hours

MAPS *Explore Yarmouth's Nature Trails*, a booklet available from the Town of Yarmouth; *Dennis*, USGS

SCENERY Chase Garden Creek, forest, salt marsh

EXPOSURE TO SUN Partial

TRAIL TRAFFIC Light

TRAIL SURFACE(S) Dirt, sand

TRAILS OPEN All year

FEES/PASSES None

FACILITIES None at trailhead; restrooms at Grays Beach

TRAIL USE

BICYCLES Trails not suitable for bicycles

DOGS Allowed on leash

HUNTING Allowed in season only in salt marsh, not in upland areas

HEALTH STATS

NUMBER OF STEPS 7,200

ESTIMATED CALORIES BURNED 343

DIRECTIONS TO TRAILHEAD

From the intersection of Route 6A and Old Church Street in Yarmouthport, marked by a flashing signal, take Old Church Street north 0.3 miles to Center Street, bear right, and go 0.2 miles to Homers Dock Road. Turn right, follow the road as it turns left after 0.1 mile, and go 0.3 miles to a roadside parking area, left. The trailhead is on the west side of the parking area.

To the parking area for a car shuttle: From the intersection of Route 6A and Old Church Street in Yarmouthport, take Route 6A west 0.4 miles to Homestead Lane. Turn right and go 0.3 miles to Kingsbury Lane. Turn right on Kingsbury Lane and go about 100 yards to a small paved parking area on the right.

WALK SUMMARY

This traverse of an important Mid-Cape conservation area encounters a variety of different habitats—forest, thickets, salt marsh—and affords visitors the chance to study the plants and animals living therein. Time your walk around low tide to avoid crossing a flooded marsh. (For a one-way walk using a car shuttle, see Directions to Trailhead, right.)

DESCRIPTION

A level sandy trail leads into a forest. After about 100 yards, a trail joins sharply from the left, and you veer right. At a junction marked by a post but no sign, turn right and wind through dense vegetation. A short path on the right leads to a bench overlooking a salt marsh. This marsh borders Chase Garden Creek, the boundary between Yarmouth and Dennis.

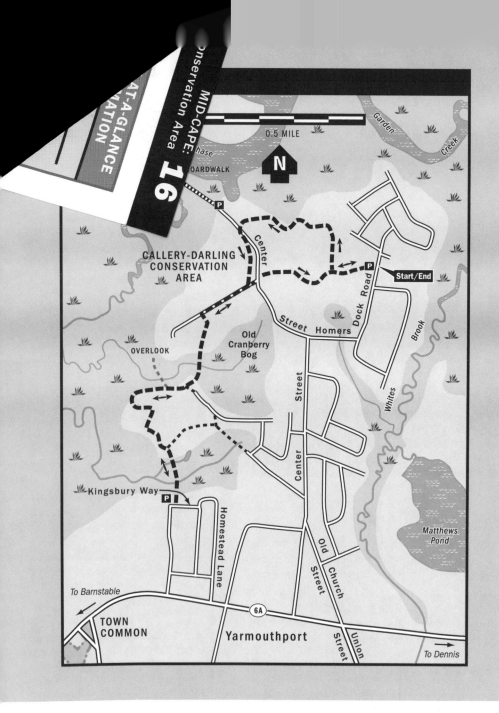

MID-CAPE: **16**
Conservation Area
AT-A-GLANCE
...ATION

0.5 MILE

N

...hase
...OARDWALK

P

CALLERY-DARLING
CONSERVATION
AREA

Center

Garden
Creek

P Start/End

Dock Road

Street Homers

Old
Cranberry
Bog

OVERLOOK

Street

Whites

Brook

Kingsbury Way **P**

Homestead Lane

Center
Street

Matthews
Pond

To Barnstable

Old
Church
Street

TOWN
COMMON

6A

Yarmouthport

Union
Street

To Dennis

Continuing another 200 feet or so, leave the woodland and enter the marsh. Follow the trail, which may be just a muddy depression in the salt hay, and step across a narrow channel. Many of the Cape's salt marshes were channeled in the past for mosquito control. Now back in a wooded area, soon reach a grassy picnic area, part of the facilities at Grays Beach. Turn left, cross the pic-

FLORA

Habitat diversity means plant diversity, and this walk passes through forest, thickets, and salt marsh. Pitch pine, white pine, black oak, white oak, black cherry, eastern red cedar, gray birch, speckled alder, quaking aspen, and horse chestnut are some of the woodland species. Arrowwood, bayberry, highbush blueberry, chokeberry, and sheep laurel form the shrubby thickets, along with poison ivy, wild grape, honeysuckle, bittersweet, greenbrier, Virginia creeper, and ferns. Marsh plants include saltwater cordgrass, salt hay, groundsel tree, marsh elder, sea lavender, glasswort, salt-spray rose, common reed, and cattail.

FAUNA

The calls of blue jays, tufted titmice, Carolina wrens, gray catbirds, mourning doves, and other songsters enliven the forest. In and above the salt marsh, look for gulls, terns, cormorants, herons, ducks, geese, and osprey. Red squirrels, smaller than their eastern gray cousins, may be active in late summer and early fall, joining other mammals such as deer, foxes, and rabbits.

nic area (seasonal restrooms on your right), and then angle right to a large paved parking area at the end of Center Street.

Grays Beach is at the mouth of Chase Garden Creek, southeast of Bass Hole, where the creek empties into Cape Cod Bay. In addition to a protected swimming area, the beach has a boat ramp, a disabled-access ramp and observation platform, and a long, wheelchair-accessible boardwalk that extends northwest over the adjoining salt marsh.

After enjoying the beach and salt marsh, walk southeast on Center Street about 100 yards from the parking area to a trailhead on the right side of the street. From there, follow a trail through a dense wooded corridor, and then across marsh via a boardwalk, about 0.1 mile to a junction beside a bench. (Take note of this junction—you will return here later.)

Turn right and emerge at a gravel parking area. Bear left, passing another bench and a map board, both on your right, and then follow a dirt-and-gravel road. Where the road begins to bend left toward Center Street, at about the 1-mile point, turn sharply right on a dirt road and head southwest along a corridor of tall trees. Continue straight past two driveways, both on the right. About 30 feet beyond the second driveway, angle left on a single-track dirt trail, as directed by a sign reading TRAIL (the road ahead is for residents only).

Now the trail traverses a dike separating a salt marsh, right, from an old cranberry bog, left. A culvert through the dike channels water from the bog into Bass Creek, which flows through the marsh to Cape Cod Bay. Back in a woodland, curve right and climb past a residential area on the left. Soon you'll merge with a dirt road by veering right. Just ahead, an overgrown dirt road on the right leads to an overlook with views of the marsh.

About 0.2 miles past the road to the overlook, you reach a junction. Turn left on a single-track trail, which follows a rolling course. At the next junction, where a trail goes left to Green Teal Way, angle right. Crossing the marsh-bordered Lone Tree Creek via a boardwalk, soon arrive at the trail's southern terminus and a parking area off Kingsbury Way. From there, retrace your route to the junction mentioned in the fourth paragraph, above.

Now veer right on a dirt trail and go about 50 feet to Center Street. Cross the street and find the trail's continuation in a tunnel of trees and shrubs. Curve left to the post-marked junction you met at the start of this walk. Go straight, then swerve left at upcoming fork to retrace your route to the parking area.

KEY AT-A-GLANCE INFORMATION

GENERAL

DISTANCE 1.2 miles

TYPE OF WALK Balloon

DIFFICULTY Easy

TIME TO WALK 1–2 hours

MAPS *Trail Guide: Historical Society of Old Yarmouth*, available at the gatehouse; *Hyannis*, USGS

SCENERY Forest, kettle pond

EXPOSURE TO SUN None

TRAIL TRAFFIC Light

TRAIL SURFACE(S) Dirt

TRAILS OPEN All year

FEES/PASSES Small donation for nonmembers

FACILITIES None

TRAIL USE

BICYCLES Not allowed

DOGS Allowed on leash

HUNTING Not allowed

HEALTH STATS

NUMBER OF STEPS 2,700

ESTIMATED CALORIES BURNED 129

DIRECTIONS TO TRAILHEAD

From the intersection of Route 6A and Willow Street in Yarmouthport, take Route 6A east 0.5 miles, to just before the post office; then turn right on a paved entrance road and go several hundred feet to a small parking area, left. (A larger parking area, for the Captain Bangs Hallet house, is just ahead.)

From the intersection of Route 6A and Union Street in Yarmouthport, take Route 6A west 0.9 miles, to just past the post office; then turn left and follow the directions above.

The trailhead is across the entrance road, just left of the gatehouse and herb garden, at a fenced dirt-and-gravel road.

Nature Trail

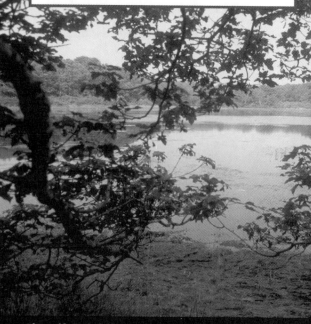

The self-guided Nature Trail passes north of Miller Pond, which can be circled on the adjoining Pond Trail.

WALK SUMMARY

Spend an hour or two exploring this small but botanically rich open space via the self-guided Nature Trail and perhaps also the Pond Trail, which circles Miller Pond. The trails pass through forest lands owned by the Historical Society of Old Yarmouth and also by Woodside Cemetery.

Boldface numbers in the description following refer to numbered markers along the trail, which are keyed to text in *Trail Guide: Historical Society of Old Yarmouth*, a pamphlet available at the gatehouse near the trailhead.

If you have time, also visit the Captain Bangs Hallet House, whose grounds feature a huge English weeping beech tree, more than 100 years old, and other exotic trees. The house, which is just uphill from the trailhead parking area, is open to the public

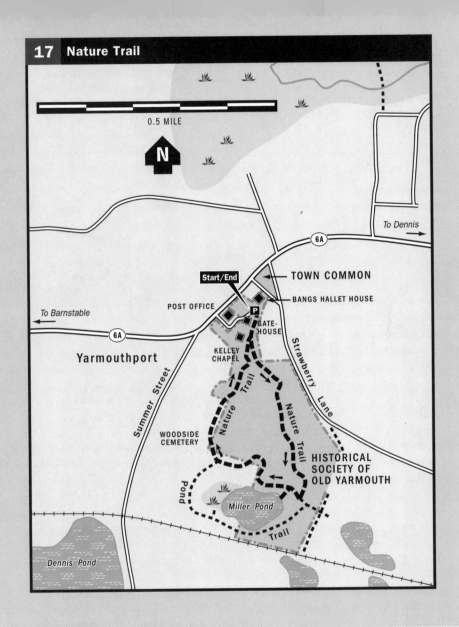

0.5 MILE

N

To Dennis →

6A

Start/End

TOWN COMMON

BANGS HALLET HOUSE

POST OFFICE

To Barnstable ←

6A

P

GATE-HOUSE

Yarmouthport

KELLEY CHAPEL

Strawberry Lane

Summer Street

Nature Trail

Nature Trail

WOODSIDE CEMETERY

HISTORICAL SOCIETY OF OLD YARMOUTH

Pond

Miller Pond

Trail

Dennis Pond

Thursday through Sunday, June to mid-October; tours are at 1, 2, and 3 p.m., groups by appointment. For more information, call (508) 362-3021.

DESCRIPTION

Follow the Nature Trail, here a dirt-and-gravel road, southwest past the gatehouse; then swing left on a single-track trail, marked with white blazes painted

FLORA	FAUNA
A combination of native and planted species makes this area rich in botanical interest. Pitch pine, white pine, black oak, white oak, eastern red cedar, black cherry, red maple, gray birch, sassafras, shadbush, American holly, yellow poplar, Norway spruce, autumn olive, and English oak are some of the trees found here. Shrubs include arrowwood, bayberry, black huckleberry, highbush blueberry, sweet pepperbush, sheep laurel, mountain laurel, and rhododendron. The dense forest provides a perfect habitat for vines such as poison ivy, Virginia creeper, honeysuckle, wild grape, and bittersweet. Check the pond for yellow pond lilies and the pond shore for Plymouth gentian.	Birds may be hard to spot in the dense forest, but listen for songs and calls of the northern cardinal, tufted titmouse, blue jay, eastern towhee, Carolina wren, and black-capped chickadee.

on trees. A tulip, or yellow, poplar, a southern species, is at the junction. Marker **1** (wooded hillside) is either missing or well hidden. After 50 feet or so, you'll come to marker **2,** left, at the base of a large English oak. Wind through a corridor of trees and shrubs to marker **3,** left, beside an overgrown pasture.

A rolling course through dense woodland brings you to marker **4** and a rest bench, both on the right. Many unofficial trails diverge from the main trail: ignore these. Curve right and climb some widely spaced steps into more open forest, mainly pines and oaks. Markers **5** and **6,** which indicate pitch pine, are to the right but hard to see. Now you crest a low rise and descend gently past a massive rhododendron to a rest bench and marker **7,** both on the left.

Climb across a hillside, passing marker **8,** right. Descend moderately, aided by steps, to a junction beside Miller Pond. Here the Pond Trail goes left, and the Nature Trail goes right. Turn right, then immediately angle left on a short trail to a rest bench and marker **9,** both beside the pond's muddy shore. Enjoy a view of the pond, then return to the main trail and go left. Marker **10** is either missing or hard to see, but what it indicates, greenbrier, is plentiful to your right.

Climb slightly to marker **11,** left, and a rest bench, right, which affords a view of the pond through a screen of trees. Now the trail curves right and continues to climb. At a low concrete barrier, turn left, passing a stand of kalmia, or mountain laurel, which produces beautiful pink or white flowers in late spring to early summer. Mountain laurel is much less common on the Cape than its cousin, sheep laurel.

In an open parklike area, reach a rest bench and markers **12** and **13,** all to the right, and then again meet the Pond Trail, left, marked by yellow blazes. (To circle the pond, which is mostly hidden from view, turn left and follow the Pond Trail to its junction with the Nature Trail on the east corner of pond. Then retrace your route on the north side of the pond to close the loop at the junction just past marker **13.** This adds about 0.75 miles to the walk.)

Turn right, pass marker **14,** and crest a low rise. Marker **15** is on your right, and just past it is a narrow, overgrown path that leads through an old clay pit, where you may find heather, wild indigo, and gray birch. The Nature Trail makes a winding descent, then levels as it passes marker **16.** After an unofficial trail joins from the right, you'll descend widely spaced dirt steps. Markers **17** (gray birch) and **18** (English oak, blue spruce, Norway spruce) are either missing or hard to see.

The Kelley Chapel, on your left, was built in 1873 in South Yarmouth and moved here in 1960. Owned by the Historical Society of Old Yarmouth, this nondenominational chapel is now used for weddings and special events. After closing the loop at the junction just past the chapel, retrace your route to the parking area.

KEY AT-A-GLANCE INFORMATION

GENERAL

DISTANCE 1.4 miles

TYPE OF WALK Loop

DIFFICULTY Easy

TIME TO WALK 1 hour or less

MAPS *Dennis*, USGS

SCENERY Cape Cod Bay, Quivett Creek, restored open fields

EXPOSURE TO SUN Full

TRAIL TRAFFIC Light

TRAIL SURFACE(S) Dirt, sand

TRAILS OPEN All year

FEES/PASSES None

FACILITIES None

TRAIL USE

BICYCLES Allowed

DOGS Allowed on leash or under voice control

HUNTING Allowed in season

HEALTH STATS

NUMBER OF STEPS 3,150

ESTIMATED CALORIES BURNED 120

DIRECTIONS TO TRAILHEAD

From the intersection of Route 6A and Route 134 in East Dennis, take Route 6A east 0.8 miles to School Street; then turn left. Go 0.1 mile to South Street, turn right, and go 0.5 miles to the end of the paved road. Continue on a single-lane, unimproved dirt road, and be alert for oncoming traffic. At 0.3 miles, stay left at a fork and go left again at the next fork. At 0.3 miles, stay right at a fork. A drive-way joins from the left at 0.5 miles; stay right at the fork just ahead. Go straight at the next 3 intersections, where roads depart left. At 0.7 miles, turn left into a dirt parking area. The trailhead is on the east corner of the parking area.

Shoreline Loop

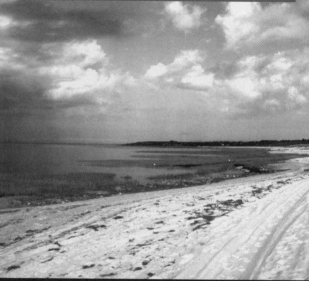

Walk at Crowes Pasture includes a stroll beside Cape Cod Bay to the mouth of Quivett Creek.

WALK SUMMARY

Crowes Pasture Conservation Area is a victory for open space in an era that has seen the building of trophy homes beside the Cape's environmentally sensitive beaches and marshes. This loop takes you through woodland, along the shore of Cape Cod Bay, beside Quivett Creek and its bordering salt marsh, and through restored open fields—wildflower-filled in late summer and fall. Time your walk to start about two or three hours after high tide; this way, you will have more room on the beach, and the sand will be firm.

Four-wheel-drive use (on beach by permit) is allowed. Hunting is allowed in season; orange hat or cap are required during hunting season.

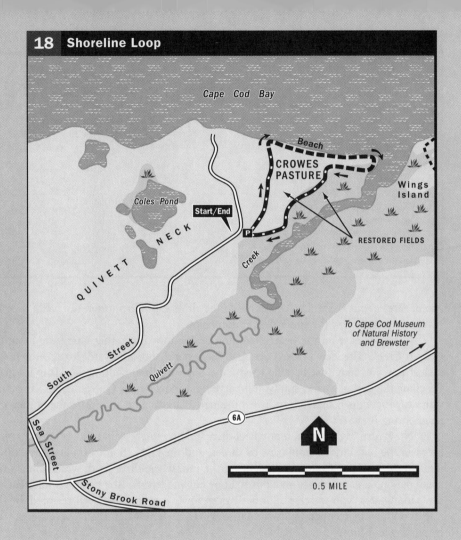

Cape Cod Bay

Beach

CROWES
PASTURE

Wings
Island

Coles Pond

Start/End

RESTORED FIELDS

QUIVETT NECK

Creek

To Cape Cod Museum
of Natural History
and Brewster

South Street

Quivett

Sea Street

6A

N

0.5 MILE

Stony Brook Road

DESCRIPTION

Walk back (west) on the dirt road 100 feet or so; then turn right on a dirt road. Passing a stone wall, right, you soon reach a fork in a sandy clearing—the road loops back on itself here. Bear left then angle left on a dirt road that winds through a wooded area to a turn-around. From here, a four-wheel-drive road (Town of Dennis permit required to drive) joins sharply from the left and goes straight to the beach on Cape Cod Bay.

Follow the four-wheel-drive road to the shore; then turn right. A rope on your right protects the sensitive dune environment. Gaps in the rope indicate places where it is OK to cross the dunes on foot—vehicles must stay along the

FLORA

The woodlands here hold pitch pine, scrub oak, black oak, white oak, black cherry, and eastern red cedar. Bordering the dirt roads are shrubs such as highbush blueberry, arrowwood, dwarf sumac, winterberry, chokeberry, and bayberry. Poison ivy, Virginia creeper, greenbrier, and honeysuckle twine through the forest.

Along the shore, look for American beach grass, beach plum, beach pea, dusty miller, seaside goldenrod, cocklebur, sea rocket, spartina, common saltwort, seabeach sandwort, and wormwood. Late summer and fall bring a gorgeous display of wildflowers, including goldenrods, asters, and blazing stars, to the restored areas of Crowes Pasture.

FAUNA

In season, geese and ducks patrol the bay, while shorebirds scamper on the sandy beach and great blue herons stalk the marsh. Overhead, barn swallows and tree swallows may be hunting insects. Gulls, crows, and blue jays often disrupt the silence with their raucous calls.

shore. After about 0.2 miles, you come to the third gap. (To shorten the walk, turn left here, and then follow the route description below.)

Continue east on the beach, strolling beside low dunes that guard the mouth of Quivett Creek. The view across Cape Cod Bay extends north toward Provincetown—on a clear day you may just be able to spy the Pilgrim Monument, some 20 miles away. Reaching the end of a sand spit, you'll curve right, now beside Quivett Creek, a twisting waterway that cuts generally southwest through a large marsh and forms the border with neighboring Brewster.

Now turn right on a four-wheel-drive road, mostly soft sand, that runs west between the bay, hidden from view by dunes, and the creek. Soon a trail over the dunes joins from the right. Continue straight on the four-wheel-drive road, which climbs to a small parking area. Here get on a dirt road by angling left. For the next 0.2 miles back to the parking area, you traverse a formerly overgrown area that has been restored, by cutting and mowing, to open fields similar to what was here when the land was kept clear by grazing and fires.

Bass River Ramble

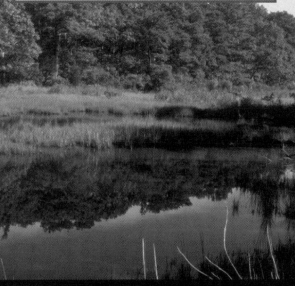

Indian Lands is a small conservation area wedged between a salt marsh, pictured here, and the Bass River.

 KEY AT-A-GLANCE INFORMATION

GENERAL

DISTANCE 1.3 miles

TYPE OF WALK Balloon

DIFFICULTY Easy

TIME TO WALK 1 hour or less

MAPS *Dennis*, USGS

SCENERY Bass River, forest, salt marsh

EXPOSURE TO SUN Partial

TRAIL TRAFFIC Moderate

TRAIL SURFACE(S) Dirt, sand

TRAILS OPEN All year

FEES/PASSES None

FACILITIES Restrooms (at Dennis town hall)

TRAIL USE

BICYCLES Allowed

DOGS Allowed on leash or under voice control

HUNTING Allowed in season

HEALTH STATS

NUMBER OF STEPS 2,925

ESTIMATED CALORIES BURNED 139

DIRECTIONS TO TRAILHEAD

From Route 6 in Dennis, take Exit 9A and follow Route 134 south 0.3 miles; then turn right on Main Street. Stay right at the next intersection (with Market Place), go 0.7 miles, and turn right into a paved parking area for the Dennis town hall. Park along the right (north) side of the parking area. The trailhead is just beside the northwest corner of the parking area.

WALK SUMMARY

This short and easy stroll, shaded for most of the way, is perfect on a warm day—but don't overlook late spring, when lady's slippers bloom, or late summer and early fall, when autumn colors enliven the salt marshes along with their bordering trees and shrubs.

DESCRIPTION

Follow a power-line access path, dirt and gravel, to four-way junction, where you turn left on a wide dirt trail. A sketch map and an INDIAN LANDS CONSERVATION AREA sign are beside the trail. Entering a forest, pass a trail joining from the right. Now you wander between two salt marshes, which are colorfully photogenic in fall. A short path departs left to

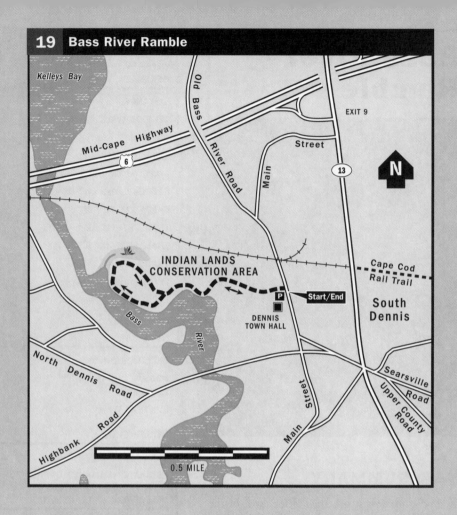

a viewpoint, and just ahead a perfectly situated rest bench overlooks the scenic Bass River.

Follow the trail as it turns right and crosses a narrow isthmus that separates river from marsh. Bear left at a fork and stroll beside the river, passing another rest bench on your right. Follow the trail as it curves right and comes to a fork; the left branch leads to a rest bench. Bear right and follow a contour across a low bluff overlooking a narrow creek that feeds the larger of the two marshes. Closing the loop, you'll cross the isthmus and retrace your route to the parking area.

FLORA

For a small area, there is rich plant diversity here. Pitch pine, white pine, black oak, white oak, red maple, black cherry, shadbush, and tupelo form the forest, complemented by highbush blueberry, black huckleberry, bayberry, scrub oak, and arrowwood. Beside the salt marsh look for groundsel tree and marsh elder, along with colorful goldenrods and asters.

Cape Cod: Lower Cape

KEY AT-A-GLANCE INFORMATION

GENERAL

DISTANCE 1.3 miles

TYPE OF WALK Balloon

DIFFICULTY Easy

TIME TO WALK 1 hour or less

MAPS *Trail Map & Guide,* available from museum; *Orleans,* USGS

SCENERY Cape Cod Bay, salt marsh

EXPOSURE TO SUN Partial

TRAIL TRAFFIC Moderate

TRAIL SURFACE(S) Dirt, sand

TRAILS OPEN All year

FEES/PASSES None

FACILITIES Natural history museum (open Wednesday–Sunday, 10 a.m.– 4 p.m.) with exhibits, library, store; restrooms (for museum visitors); wild-flower garden

TRAIL USE

BICYCLES Not allowed

DOGS Allowed on leash

HUNTING Not allowed

HEALTH STATS

NUMBER OF STEPS 2,925

ESTIMATED CALORIES BURNED 139

DIRECTIONS TO TRAILHEAD

From the intersection of Route 6A and Route 137 in Brewster, take Route 6A west 1.6 miles; then turn right into a large gravel parking area for the Cape Cod Museum of Natural History. The trailhead is on the west corner of the parking area, beside the museum entrance.

John Wing Trail

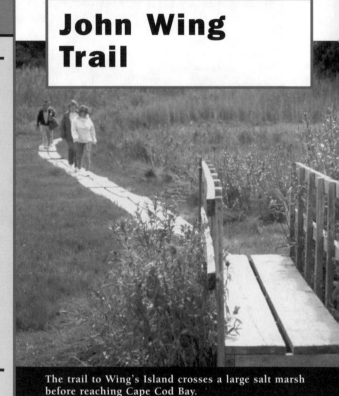

The trail to Wing's Island crosses a large salt marsh before reaching Cape Cod Bay.

WALK SUMMARY

Follow the John Wing Trail to Wing's Island, a low wooded hill bordered by salt marsh and Cape Cod Bay, and imagine yourself transported back in time. Early settlers harvested salt hay from the marshes and produced salt through evaporation of seawater. Agriculture and fires created large open fields and meadows, which were home to many species of birds and butterflies. A five-year restoration project, begun in 2004, is converting several of Wing's Island's woodlands to clearings and will hopefully return some of the species long missing from the area, thus setting back the ecological clock to an earlier era. (If you have time, you can combine this walk with a short stroll on the Lee Baldwin Trail, which leaves from the southeast corner of a parking area just across Route 6A from the museum.)

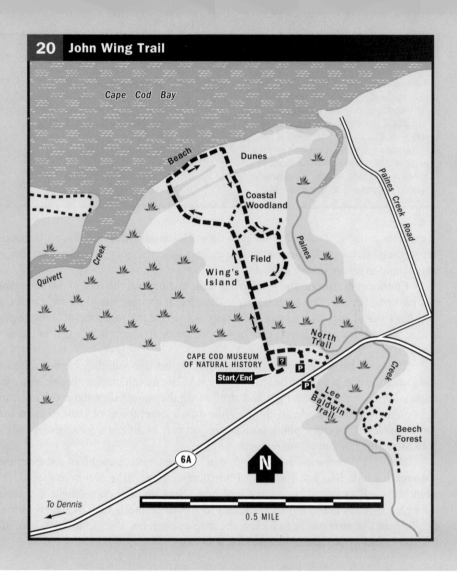

DESCRIPTION

The John Wing Trail starts as a short boardwalk that leads northwest to a dirt trail bordered by trees and shrubs. Cross a paved driveway; then pass the North Trail, which joins from the right. Soon you leave the woods behind and reach a boardwalk across the salt marsh separating Wing's Island (aka Wing Island and Wings Island) from the mainland. Many of the Cape's salt marshes have straight, narrow channels in them; these were dug in the past for mosquito control. Today, nesting boxes for birds are used to attract mosquito-eating predators.

Now on a sandy path, pass a trail on your right, signed for the John Wing monument, which you will visit later. Climb gently through forest to a junction

FLORA	FAUNA
Many plants are berry producers—among those here are black cherry, highbush blueberry, arrowwood, beach plum, bayberry, chokeberry, poison ivy, greenbrier, bittersweet, wild grape, and Virginia creeper. Pitch pine, scrub oak, black oak, dwarf chestnut oak, and eastern red cedar dominate the woodlands, whereas the salt marsh is home to saltwater cordgrass, salt hay, glasswort, sea lavender, groundsel tree, and marsh elder.	Gulls, terns, and shorebirds frequent the beach, especially near the mouths of Quivett Creek and Stony Brook. In autumn, sea ducks congregate just offshore or pass by in large flocks. Wooded Wing's Island is home to black-capped chickadees, blue jays, and other woodland birds.

where a short trail to a solar calendar goes right. This installation, built by Jeff Thibodeau, marks the position of the sun on equinoxes and solstices. Solar calendars like this one were common among native cultures.

Continue straight on the John Wing Trail; just beyond the trail to the solar calendar, pass another trail that branches right. Veer left at an upcoming fork and, with Cape Cod Bay in view, approach a large salt marsh. Stay left at the next fork and cross a plank bridge over a branch of Quivett Creek. A short, sandy trek now brings you to the shore of the bay.

The main branch of Quivett Creek, which forms the boundary between Brewster and Dennis, empties into the bay just to your left. The mouth of Stony Brook, also called Paine's Creek, is right. Turn right and stroll along the shore. After about 0.1 mile, turn right on a trail going southeast through low dunes. Several sets of wooden steps bring you to an elevated vantage point, from where you may be able to spy Provincetown's Pilgrim Monument, about 20 miles north.

Now in a dense woodland of stout, wind-pruned pines, pass a trail going right and soon reach a fork. Bear left, come to a T-junction, and turn right. Southern species, such as hickory and sassafras, border the trail here. Now the trail curves right and cruises through a shrubby corridor. Just ahead is a memorial honoring John Wing, an early settler. Beyond the memorial, you'll close the loop at the John Wing Trail. From here, turn left and retrace your route to the parking area.

Cliff and Little Cliff Ponds

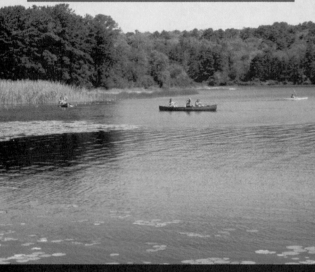

Little Cliff Pond is a tranquil oasis in the heart of Nickerson State Park.

ⓘ KEY AT-A-GLANCE INFORMATION

GENERAL

DISTANCE 3.9 miles

TYPE OF WALK Loop

DIFFICULTY Moderate

TIME TO WALK 2–3 hours

MAPS Handout from information booth; *Orleans*, USGS

SCENERY Forest, kettle ponds

EXPOSURE TO SUN Partial

TRAIL TRAFFIC Moderate

TRAIL SURFACE(S) Dirt, sand

TRAILS OPEN All year

FEES/PASSES None

FACILITIES Toilets (seasonal) at the trailhead; near the park entrance are restrooms (seasonal), nature center (seasonal), and phone; there is a park store (seasonal) on Deer Park Road.

TRAIL USE

BICYCLES Not on single-track trails (including part of this route) in summer

DOGS Allowed on leash

HUNTING Not allowed

HEALTH STATS

NUMBER OF STEPS 8,775

ESTIMATED CALORIES BURNED 419

DIRECTIONS TO TRAILHEAD

From Route 6 northbound in Orleans, take Exit 12 to Route 6A. Turn left, go 1.5 miles, and then turn left into Nickerson State Park. There is a large parking area on the right with restrooms and an information booth (both seasonal). Continue past the parking area, now on Flax Pond Road. At 0.3 miles Flax Pond Road turns left and Deer Park Road goes straight. Turn left and go another 1.1 mile to the parking area for Cliff and Little Cliff ponds.

From Route 6 southbound in Orleans, take Exit 12 to Route 6A. Turn right, go 1.4 miles, and then turn left into the Nickerson State Park. Now follow the directions above.

WALK SUMMARY

Nickerson State Park is one of the Cape's gems, providing year-round public access to about 1,900 acres of open space. More than 400 seasonal campsites beckon, along with trails for walking, bicycling, horseback riding, and even cross-country skiing. Several large kettle ponds offer opportunities for swimming, nonmotorized boating, and fishing. This scenic loop circles most of Little Cliff Pond and then explores the forested shoreline of much larger Cliff Pond. If water levels are high, there are inland trails through the woods that border each pond, but some of these trails may be overgrown. Because of the state park's popularity, this walk is best done during the off-season.

Note: A fire in the summer of 2005 destroyed the former entrance station; plans to rebuild are

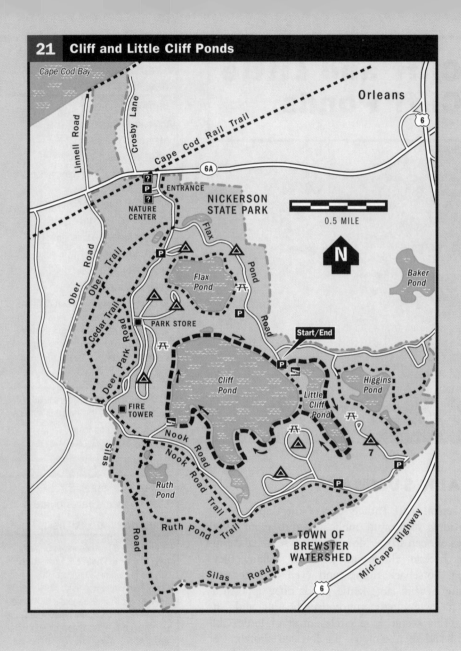

uncertain. There is currently a staffed information booth with maps and brochures (seasonal), located on the north side of the parking area immediately to your right as you first enter the park.

FLORA	FAUNA
Trees here include pitch pine, black oak, white oak, black cherry, red maple, black locust, bigtooth aspen, hickory, and sassafras. Joining them are shrubs such as alder, highbush blueberry, sweet pepperbush, bayberry, black huckleberry, and hazelnut. Ground cover includes bearberry, checkerberry, greenbrier, and poison ivy. Beside Little Cliff Pond, look for Plymouth gentian—gorgeous pink (sometimes white) flowers with bright yellow centers. Pickerelweed and white water lilies grow in the pond itself.	Cormorants and Canada geese may be floating in the ponds. Spotted sandpipers, one of the few shorebirds to favor fresh water, are present during the summer. Osprey cruise overhead and sometimes dive for fish. Eastern kingbirds, nuthatches, and ovenbirds are some of the forest species to look and listen for. Tracks in mud may reveal the usually nocturnal journeys of deer, coyote, skunks, foxes, or raccoons.

DESCRIPTION

The trailhead is just southeast of the parking area, at the boat ramp for Little Cliff Pond. Just left of the boat ramp, find a faint trail that skirts Little Cliff Pond, a narrow body of water that was probably once part of Cliff Pond, its larger neighbor to the west. The overgrown and possibly muddy trail threads its way between the pond's sandy shoreline on the right and a forest to your left. The water level of kettle ponds rises with rainfall and falls with evaporation, so the width of the land between forest and pond varies. (If the pond shore is flooded, use the upland trail located several hundred feet northwest of the boat ramp, on the east side of Flax Pond Road.)

At the pond's southeast end, bear right across a sandy beach, with a freshwater marsh on your left, and continue your clockwise circuit of the pond. Just before reaching a stand of common reeds, you'll come to a path used by canoeists and kayakers to portage their boats from Little Cliff Pond to Cliff Pond. Veer left and climb a low rise to a junction. Here a trail goes left into a wooded area and soon becomes overgrown with greenbrier and poison ivy. Continue straight and descend to one of Cliff Pond's lovely sandy beaches. In summer this is the site of the Brewster Day Camp and Jack's Boat Rentals. (To shorten the walk, turn right and follow the shoreline or a wooded path north, then northwest, to the parking area.)

Now begin a clockwise circuit of Cliff Pond, staying along the shoreline. Rocks and stones underfoot are clues to the formation of the Cape's landscape, which consists mostly of glacial moraines and outwash plains. Follow the shoreline as it bends left into a cove and comes to another sandy beach. Curve right, cross the beach, and then contour at pond level around a steep, wooded hillside that juts northwest into the pond. The trail bends abruptly left and takes you into another, larger, cove.

When you reach a beach, at about the 2-mile point, turn right and follow a narrow strip of sand between Cliff Pond, right, and a large marsh, left. At the beach's far end, find a wide path and climb gently to a fork. Bear right and traverse a steep slope, which drops to the pond. Now follow a winding, rolling course that soon brings you to a four-way junction. Go straight, ignoring various side paths, and soon merge with a trail joining sharply from the left.

Just ahead, you'll pass a narrow, overgrown path angling right, to a beach. Continue straight and, at the next junction, turn right on a trail that leads to a parking area for a public boat landing. Passing a paved boat ramp and a wooden boardwalk, both right, continue along the pond's shore, with a marsh to your left. Follow the shoreline north to a sandy beach dotted with large glacial boulders.

Once past the beach, find a trail that goes just left of a grove of trees and shrubs growing at the water's edge. Now the trail wanders amid stunted pines, with a small marsh to your left. When you reach an open beach with PRIVATE PROPERTY signs on your left, stay along the shoreline to find the continuation of the trail, which is marked with a Cape Cod Pathways sign and blue triangles with a hiking symbol. The trail skirts the pond at the foot of a steep hillside that rises left. Walk through a narrow corridor of dense vegetation and then angle left and climb steeply to a pine forest.

After cresting the hillside, bear right and walk parallel to the pond shore. With private property to the left, descend gently and follow a narrow track perched precariously above the pond. Passing a small beach, which is on the right, soon angle left to the parking area.

Silas Road

GENERAL

DISTANCE 4 miles

TYPE OF WALK Loop

DIFFICULTY Moderate

TIME TO WALK 2–3 hours

MAPS Handout from information booth; *Orleans*, USGS

SCENERY Forest

EXPOSURE TO SUN Partial

TRAIL TRAFFIC Light

TRAIL SURFACE(S) Dirt, pavement, sand

TRAILS OPEN All year

FEES/PASSES None

FACILITIES None at the trailhead; near the entrance are restrooms (seasonal), nature center (seasonal), and phone; park store (seasonal) on Deer Park Road

TRAIL USE

BICYCLES On dirt roads and bike trails; single-track trails not suitable for bicycles

DOGS Allowed on leash

HUNTING Not allowed

HEALTH STATS

NUMBER OF STEPS 9,000

ESTIMATED CALORIES BURNED 429

DIRECTIONS TO TRAILHEAD

From Route 6 northbound in Orleans, take Exit 12 to Route 6A. Turn left, go 1.5 miles, and turn left into Nickerson State Park. At right are restrooms and an information booth (seasonal). Continue past this area, now on Flax Pond Road. At 0.3 miles Flax Pond Road turns left and Deer Park Road goes straight. Take Deer Park Road 1.2 miles to where the road turns left and becomes Nook Road. Go 0.3 miles on Nook Road, and turn left on a dirt road to the Cliff Pond boat landing. Park beside the road or at the end of the road.

From Route 6 southbound in Orleans, take Exit 12 to Route 6A. Turn right, go 1.4 miles, and turn left into the Nickerson State Park. Now follow directions above.

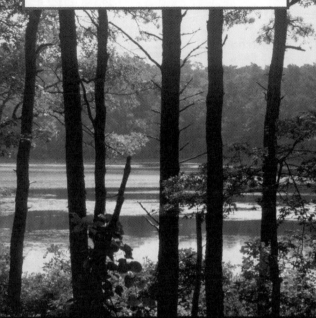

Ruth Pond Trail skirts its namesake pond on the way to Silas Road.

WALK SUMMARY

The route combines a sunny ramble on a dirt road with a shady stroll on a paved bike trail. A wide variety of trees and shrubs will keep botanical enthusiasts busy, and birders should bring binoculars. Because of the state park's popularity and the route's exposure to sun, this walk is best done during the off-season. *Note:* A fire in the summer of 2005 destroyed the former entrance station; plans to rebuild are uncertain. There is currently a staffed information booth (seasonal) with brochures and maps located on the north side of the parking area immediately to your right as you first enter the park.

DESCRIPTION

The trailhead is at the bike trail on the southwest side of Nook Road, several hundred feet northwest of

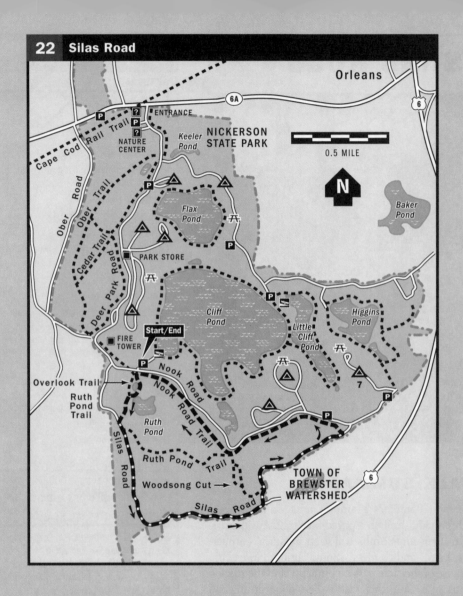

the dirt road to the Cliff Pond boat landing. Two paved bike trails, the Ruth Pond Trail and the Nook Road Trail, depart from the trailhead just beyond a brown metal gate. To begin, angle slightly right on the Ruth Pond Trail and in about 100 yards reach a fork with the Overlook Trail. Remain on the Ruth Pond Trail by veering left. With Ruth Pond in view to the left, climb moderately to meet the Overlook Trail, which joins sharply from the right.

Veer left and pass a dirt path heading left. Beyond Ruth Pond, the bike trail crests a rise, descends slightly, and skirts Silas Road, which is immediately right. Join Silas Road—a dirt road closed to vehicles—by angling right and turning left. Follow Silas Road south, passing a brown metal gate and a wide path (a dirt road shown on some maps as Ruth Pond Road), which are both left.

The road runs straight for a while, rising on a gentle grade. Along the way, a number of paths diverge from Silas Road: ignore these. At about the 0.8-mile point, a trail departs right and your road angles slightly left, then right. After a level stretch, descend over rocky and eroded ground. After another level stretch, Silas Road angles left and climbs moderately, passing a trail on the left, to meet a dirt road joining from the right (not on the map).

Turn left to stay on Silas Road. After about 100 feet, a trail departs left and another goes right. Continue straight; just before entering the signed Town of Brewster watershed, angle left to stay on Silas Road, here a narrow track strewn with rocks. Climb gently to a junction, at about the 1.8-mile point, with Woodsong Cut on the left. (To shorten the walk, turn left on Woodsong Cut, bear right at a T-junction and left at the next junction. At the paved Nook Road Trail [bike trail], turn left and follow the route description below.)

Beyond the junction, Silas Road rises moderately over rough and rocky ground. Soon the grade eases and you pass a short dirt road to a clearing, which is left. Curve left and descend to a fork. Angle left and in about 50 feet join Nook Road Trail (paved bike trail) by turning left. Enjoy a westward stroll parallel to and just south of Nook Road. After about 0.1 mile, pass a trail on the left and then a short path to Nook Road, which is right. On a lengthy course, pass a parking area and two campgrounds, which are across Nook Road.

At about the 3.1-mile point, a dirt road (not on the map) joins from the left and continues a short distance to Nook Road. The bike trail veers left, climbs, and then descends. After about 100 yards, the bike trail nearly meets a wide dirt path (Ruth Pond Road) just to the right. Ahead about 200 feet, Woodsong Cut veers left through the woods but continue straight on the paved trail. After about 250 feet, at a four-way junction, the wide dirt path (Ruth Pond Road) joins sharply from the right and also angles left.

Keep straight and in about 50 feet reach a junction at about the 3.3-mile point. Here the paved bike trails diverge—Ruth Pond Trail to the left, Nook Road Trail straight. Go straight. Just before reaching the trailhead, pass a four-way junction, where a trail leads left and a short trail goes right to a parking area beside Nook Road. Continue a short distance to the trailhead.

KEY AT-A-GLANCE INFORMATION

GENERAL

DISTANCE 2.5 miles

TYPE OF WALK Balloon

DIFFICULTY Moderate

TIME TO WALK 1–2 hours

MAPS *Punkhorn Parklands Calf Field Pond Trails*, download from town Web site; *The Punkhorn Parklands Trail Guide,* Cape Cod Pathways, available at Brewster Town Offices; *Harwich*, USGS

SCENERY Forest, kettle ponds, wetlands

EXPOSURE TO SUN None

TRAIL TRAFFIC Light

TRAIL SURFACE(S) Dirt, sand

TRAILS OPEN All year

FEES/PASSES None

FACILITIES None

TRAIL USE

BICYCLES Not allowed on single-track trails, including part of this route

DOGS Allowed on leash

HUNTING Not allowed

HEALTH STATS

NUMBER OF STEPS 5,625

ESTIMATED CALORIES BURNED 268

DIRECTIONS TO TRAILHEAD

From the intersection of Route 6A and Stony Brook Road in West Brewster, marked by a flashing yellow traffic signal, take Stony Brook Road southwest 0.6 miles to Run Hill Road. Turn left and drive 1.3 miles to a dirt parking area, left. The trailhead is on the northwest corner of the parking area.

Calf Field Pond

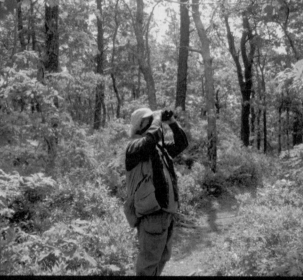

Punkhorn Parklands is a great place to learn how to identify birds by sight and sound.

WALK SUMMARY

Punkhorn is a local term whose meaning is unclear—a 1747 deed called the area "Sepunkhorn," and the shortened version is used to imply a boggy landscape, or perhaps simply "the boondocks." Whatever the definition, this 835-acre wilderness, home to dense forests, kettle ponds, and freshwater wetlands, is a walker's paradise. This invigorating route explores the Punkhorn's densely forested northeast corner and visits three small kettle ponds and their neighboring wetlands.

DESCRIPTION

From the trailhead, walk right (northeast) on Run Hill Road for about 100 yards, passing an entrance road, on the right, to the Deerfield housing development. Just beyond is a trail marked with a

23   Calf Field Pond

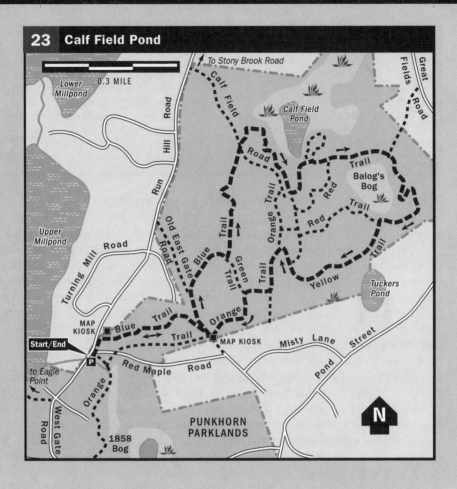

To Stony Brook Road

Lower Millpond

0.3 MILE

Calf Field Pond

Great Fields Road

Hill Road

Calf Field Road

Run Road

Upper Millpond

Turning Mill Road

Old East Gate Road

Blue Trail

Green Trail

Orange Trail

Orange Trail

Red Trail

Red Trail

Balog's Bog

Yellow Trail

Tuckers Pond

MAP KIOSK

Blue Trail

Orange Trail

Blue Trail

MAP KIOSK

Misty Lane

Street

Start/End

to Eagle Point

Red Maple Road

Pond

Orange

West Gate Road

1858 Bog

PUNKHORN PARKLANDS

N

PUNKHORN PARKLANDS CONSERVATION AREA sign and two boulders that block motor-vehicle access. As you turn right onto the Blue Trail, pass a map kiosk, a welcome feature in an area crisscrossed with a confusing array of dirt roads, paths, and trails. (In places, arrows on trail posts or colored markers on trees aid navigation, but other signage here is generally nonexistent.)

Follow the narrow sandy path through forest to a T-junction (not shown on the map); then turn left to stay on the Blue Trail. Gently gaining elevation, curve right and soon pass an unofficial trail that goes left. Now on a level course, reach a fork and bear right. Just ahead, you'll arrive at a five-way junction. The Blue Trail merges with Old East Gate Road, a dirt track that joins sharply from the left and continues straight toward residential area. The Orange Trail goes left and right. There is a map kiosk on the right. Turn sharply left on Old East Gate Road, which is the continuation of the Blue Trail.

After a dirt road joins from the left, angle right onto a single-track trail. Descend gently to a clearing, where an unofficial trail departs left. You jog right,

FLORA	FAUNA
Many of the Cape's common trees live here, including pitch pine, black oak, black cherry, red maple, and eastern red cedar. Look also for white pine, gray birch, American beech, and sassafras. Shrubs such as black huckleberry, bayberry, highbush blueberry, chokeberry, sweet pepperbush, arrowwood, and hazelnut adorn the forest.	A dense forest with limited visibility is a good place to practice "birding by ear," so listen for blue jays, white-breasted nuthatches, downy woodpeckers, gray catbirds, great-crested flycatchers, black-capped chickadees, and various warblers.

then left, and now climb on a gentle grade to a T-junction. Turn left, passing a pit that may have been a quarry for granite boulders, which were commonly used to make jetties in Cape Cod Bay—on one map, the dirt road to this pit is named Quarry Road.

After following Quarry Road for about 100 feet, veer right onto a trail as directed by an arrow on a tree. Now make a curvy climb, crest a rise, and then descend the log-crossed, winding trail. Turning sharply left to stay on the Blue Trail, crest another rise and then drop to a four-way junction with unsigned Calf Field Road. Cross the dirt road and continue descending on the Blue Trail, veering right at a fork, and enter a magical stand of American beech. These trees have shallow roots that suck nutrients from the soil; this explains the relatively barren forest floor here.

Now climb and curve right to join Calf Field Road, here part of the Blue Trail. Turn left to reach a four-way junction. Here the Orange Trail goes straight and also right, but turn left to stay on the Blue Trail. After about 100 yards, where a faint trail goes right, turn left again. Pass a closed trail, on your left, and then arrive at a junction marking the start of a small loop that the Blue Trail makes southeast of Calf Field Pond. (To visit the pond, turn left.)

Continue straight and then wind uphill to an easily missed junction. Here the Blue Trail veers sharply left, but you go straight, now on the Green Trail. Soon merge with the Red Trail, which joins sharply from the right and, just ahead, meet a poorly signed fork. Angle right to stay on the Red Trail, which circles a freshwater marsh southeast of Calf Field Pond. The marsh surrounds a wetland known as Balog's Bog. Several closed trails join from the left as you make a clockwise circuit of the marsh.

At another poorly signed junction, turn sharply left to stay on the Red Trail. Passing a closed trail, left, switchback right, climb, and descend to a junction. Here the Red Trail goes right, but you should opt for the Yellow Trail by going straight. Following a creek, on the right, that connects with Balog's Pond, climb slightly to a junction, where a short trail goes left to an overlook of the next pond south, a lovely body of water called Tuckers Pond.

Continuing straight, soon reach the next junction, where you'll turn right to stay on the Yellow Trail. A winding, rolling course takes you past an unofficial trail, left, and a closed trail, right. Now the Yellow Trail ends at a junction, where the Orange Trail goes straight and also sharply left. Turning left, climb gently, staying on the Orange Trail by veering right at the next junction, where an unofficial trail goes straight.

Having arrived at a T-junction—Green Trail right, Orange Trail left—turn left, soon passing two unofficial trails, one going left to a housing development, the other going right. Continue straight to close the loop at the five-way junction. Turn right on the Blue Trail (not sharply right on Old East Gate Road) and retrace your route to the parking area.

Eagle Point

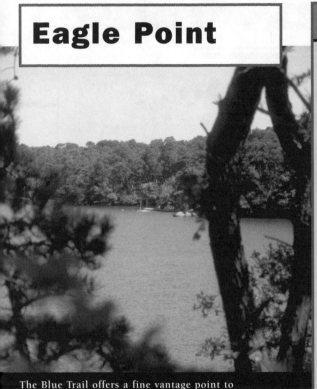

The Blue Trail offers a fine vantage point to view Upper Millpond.

GENE

DISTA

TYPE

DIFFI

TIME TO WALK 1 hour or less

MAPS *Punkhorn Parklands Eagle Point Trails,* download from town Web site; *The Punkhorn Parklands Trail Guide,* Cape Cod Pathways, available at Brewster Town Offices; *Harwich,* USGS

SCENERY Forest, kettle ponds

EXPOSURE TO SUN None

TRAIL TRAFFIC Light

TRAIL SURFACE(S) Dirt

TRAILS OPEN All year

FEES/PASSES None

FACILITIES None

TRAIL USE

BICYCLES Not allowed on single-track trails, including part of this route

DOGS Allowed on leash

HUNTING Not allowed

HEALTH STATS

NUMBER OF STEPS 1,800

ESTIMATED CALORIES BURNED 86

DIRECTIONS TO TRAILHEAD

From the intersection of Route 6A and Stony Brook Road in West Brewster, marked by a flashing yellow traffic signal, take Stony Brook Road southwest 0.6 miles to Run Hill Road. Turn left and drive 1.3 miles to a dirt parking area, left. The trailhead is on the northwest corner of the parking area.

WALK SUMMARY

This short but scenic ramble explores a hilly, densely forested part of the Punkhorn that borders Upper Millpond. Several fine vantage points along the way afford vistas of the pond, one of three linked kettle ponds that form the headwaters of Stony Brook, which flows north to Cape Cod Bay.

DESCRIPTION

To begin, walk left (southwest) on Run Hill Road for about 200 feet to a five-way junction beside the Town of Brewster water-filtration facility, which is on your left. A road leading to a boat landing on Upper Millpond goes right. Angle right on the Blue Trail, a dirt single-track trail also called the Eagle Point Trail. After about 100 feet, an unofficial trail

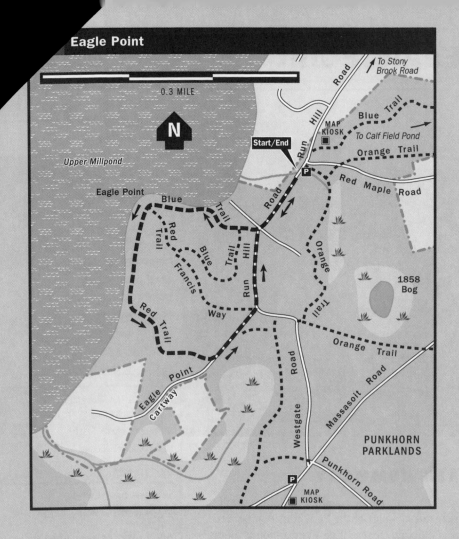

0.3 MILE

N

Upper Millpond

Eagle Point

Blue Trail

Red Trail

Blue Trail

Francis Way

Run Hill

Red Trail

Eagle Point Cartway

Start/End

To Stony Brook Road

Run Hill Road

MAP KIOSK

Blue Trail

To Calf Field Pond

Orange Trail

Red Maple Road

Orange Trail

1858 Bog

Orange Trail

Road

Westgate Road

Massasoit Road

PUNKHORN PARKLANDS

Punkhorn Road

MAP KIOSK

departs right, but you'll continue straight. The trail then crests a low rise, curves left, and descends.

At the next junction, stay straight on the Blue Trail and follow it through a narrow corridor of shrubs and trees. A freshwater marsh is to your left. Soon you'll glimpse Upper Millpond, largest of the Punkhorn's ponds. This pond and Walkers Pond, its neighbor to the southwest, are favorite canoe and kayak spots. Alewives, also called herring, swim up Stony Brook to spawn in the ponds. A historic mill graces the brook's banks on Stony Brook Road not far from here. Waterfowl, ospreys, and even bald eagles visit the ponds.

Cross a short boardwalk over a creek joining the marsh, left, with Upper Millpond, right. After passing an unofficial trail, left, climb moderately on granite

FLORA	FAUNA
Bordering Upper Millpond is a dense forest of pitch pine, black oak, white oak, black cherry, red maple, sassafras, hickory, tupelo, and American beech. Shrubs include sweet pepperbush, chokeberry, highbush blueberry, arrowwood, wild raisin, black huckleberry, scrub oak, and sheep laurel. Poison ivy and greenbrier wait for the unwary just off the trail.	Keep a sharp ear out for forest birds such as black-capped chickadees, white-breasted nuthatches, gray catbirds, and blue jays. In fall, Upper Millpond hosts flotillas of migratory waterfowl. Bald eagles are also possible visitors.

steps. Atop a hill, the trail forks, with the right-hand branch leading to a beautifully situated rest bench that commands a fine view of Upper Millpond. After the fork's branches rejoin, descend to a four-way junction. Here the Blue Trail goes left, but you go straight on the Red Trail. (The trail angling right soon merges with the Red Trail.)

Descending and then climbing, soon reach the next fork and again stay right, passing another rest bench. As you continue to gain elevation, the fork's other branch merges from the left. Descend to yet another fork and stay on the Red Trail by angling left (the right-hand branch soon rejoins). Granite steps aid your moderate descent. Stay right at the next fork as directed by a sign, and enjoy strolling through a light-dappled grove of American beech.

Upon reaching a T-junction with Eagle Point Cartway, a dirt-and-gravel road, turn left. Pass Francis Way, a dirt road on your left blocked by boulders, and Westgate Road, a dirt road joining from the right; then curve left, now on Run Hill Road. Follow this dirt road north to close the loop; then continue straight to the parking area.

Grand Tour

GENERAL

DISTANCE 5.6 miles

TYPE OF WALK Balloon

DIFFICULTY Difficult

TIME TO WALK 3–4 hours

MAPS *The Punkhorn Parklands Trail Guide*, Cape Cod Pathways, available at Brewster Town Offices; *Harwich*, USGS

SCENERY Forest, kettle ponds

EXPOSURE TO SUN None

TRAIL TRAFFIC Light

TRAIL SURFACE(S) Dirt

TRAILS OPEN All year

FEES/PASSES None

FACILITIES None

TRAIL USE

BICYCLES Not allowed on single-track trails, including part of this route

DOGS Allowed on leash

HUNTING Not allowed

HEALTH STATS

NUMBER OF STEPS 12,600

ESTIMATED CALORIES BURNED 600

DIRECTIONS

From the intersection of Route 6A and Stony Brook Road in West Brewster, marked by a flashing yellow traffic signal, take Stony Brook Road southwest 0.6 miles to Run Hill Road. Turn left and drive 1.3 miles to a dirt parking area, left. The trailhead is on the northwest corner of the parking area.

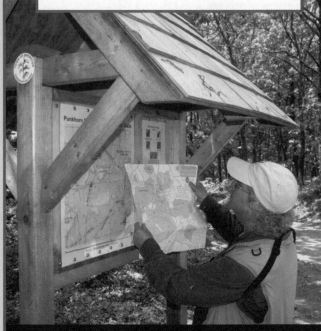

Map kiosks help visitors navigate the Punkhorn's complex network of roads and trails.

WALK SUMMARY

The Punkhorn has seen many uses since the glaciers that formed the landscape retreated. Native Americans lived here and took advantage of the fish-rich ponds and other resources. Settlers in the 18th century cut the forest and grazed sheep in the resulting meadows. The 19th century brought a cranberry industry to the area's bogs, and in the early 1900s granite for jetties was quarried near Calf Field Pond. Today, however, the Punkhorn Parklands are a place to commune with nature and enjoy the Cape's rich biodiversity. This "grand tour" visits a variety of habitats, including the area's two largest kettle ponds, a freshwater marsh, and a serene forest.

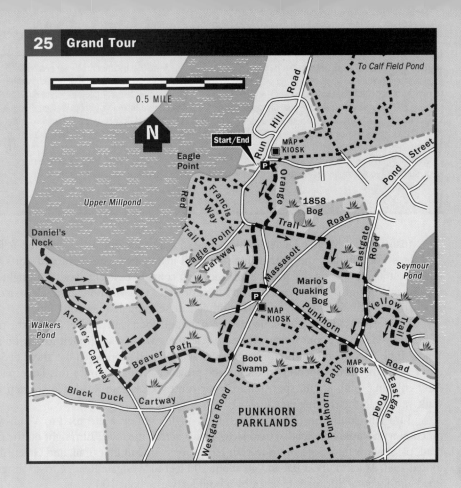

Within the map:

0.5 MILE

N

To Calf Field Pond

Run Hill Road

Start/End

MAP KIOSK

Eagle Point

Orange Trail

Pond Street

Upper Millpond

Red Trail

Francis Way

1858 Bog

Road

Daniel's Neck

Eagle Point Cartway

Massasoit

Eastgate Road

Seymour Pond

Mario's Quaking Bog

MAP KIOSK

Punkhorn

Yellow Trail

Archie's Cartway

Walkers Pond

Beaver Path

Boot Swamp

MAP KIOSK

Road

Black Duck Cartway

Westgate Road

Punkhorn Path

Eastgate Road

PUNKHORN PARKLANDS

DESCRIPTION

From the trailhead, go right (northeast) on Run Hill Road for a few feet; then turn right on a dirt road and skirt the north side of the parking area. After about 100 yards the road ends—from here, follow the Orange Trail, a dirt path that goes between two boulders and into a forest. After several hundred feet, reach a dirt road adjacent to the Town of Brewster water-filtration facility. Turn left, then immediately veer left onto the continuation of the Orange Trail.

Where a trail goes left, bear right through a junglelike corridor of trees and shrubs. A rolling, rocky course brings you to a T-junction with an overgrown dirt road. Turn left, still on the Orange Trail, and enjoy a level stroll to Massasoit Road. Cross the dirt road and then continue on the Orange Trail. Where a trail joins sharply from the left, veer right, soon passing another trail on your left, and then descend on a gentle grade through a fern-filled forest.

Just north of Mario's Quaking Bog, come to a four-way junction. Here the Yellow Trail joins from the left; the Orange Trail, not well maintained, goes right and skirts the bog. Go straight, now on the Yellow Trail, and soon come to Eastgate Road. Turn right on the dirt road, climb gently over a rise, and then descend to a junction. Turn left on a dirt road, still the Yellow Trail, and follow a winding course through a beautiful forest.

Where a closed trail goes straight, turn right and soon gain a ridge. Follow the trail as it zigzags down to a four-way junction in a clearing, where you turn left to stay on the Yellow Trail. Pass the other end of the closed trail, left, and soon reach the shore of Seymour Pond. A narrow opening in the foliage provides a window onto this large pond. After enjoying this tranquil spot, retrace your route to Eastgate Road. (To shorten the walk, retrace to the parking area.)

Turn left (south) on Eastgate Road; then angle right on a dirt road to a four-way junction with Punkhorn Road; a map kiosk is just across the road. Turn right on the dirt road, passing two junctions, both to your left—Green Trail to Blue Trail, and Green Trail to Red Trail. At a fork, bear left and go about 100 feet to Westgate Road. Cross Westgate Road and follow a dirt road, blocked by a boulder, west about 100 yards.

Just before the road begins a loop, veer right on a single-track trail. Go about 100 feet to meet a trail that runs parallel to and just west of Westgate Road. Turn sharply left, follow the trail about 40 feet to a fork, and stay left (the fork's branches soon rejoin). Now traverse a hillside of American beech, with a freshwater marsh downhill and right.

When you reach a dirt road—a brown metal gate is right—cross it and regain the single-track trail, which soon curves left to meet Westgate Road. Turn right and go about 100 feet to Beaver Path, a dirt road blocked by a boulder. Angle right on the road and descend gently to cross a culvert holding the Punkhorn River, which flows northward to Upper Millpond. An extensive freshwater marsh is on the right. Climb on a gentle grade, passing several trails branching from the road, and join Archie's Cartway, a dirt road onto which you turn right.

Soon a trail that you will use later joins on the right. Walk through a small housing development; then follow the road as it winds through a forest bordering Walkers Pond, which is on the left. Where Archie's Cartway swings to the right, branch left on a dirt road to Captain Daniel's Neck, a peninsula that separates Walkers Pond from Upper Millpond. Where the dirt road ends at some boulders, follow a grassy path that soon swings right and enters a shady alley of trees and shrubs.

A clearing marks a former homesite, now overrun with berry vines. A narrow path leads left, beside Upper Millpond, but it soon becomes too overgrown to follow. Enjoy the view of the peaceful pond, a picnic, or perhaps a swim; then retrace your route to Archie's Cartway and turn left. The road climbs moderately, levels, and then reaches a junction, right, with a single-track trail. Angle right on the trail, go about 100 yards to the next junction, and turn left.

Soon you pass a dirt road, left, leading to a house. Your trail winds through dense forest, with Upper Millpond barely visible through the trees on your left. Where paths diverge—first left, then right—you go straight. When you regain Archie's Cartway at a T-junction, turn left and retrace your route about 100 yards to Beaver Path. Angle left and retrace your route to Westgate Road. Turn left and retrace your route about 100 feet to the single-track trail that parallels Westgate Road.

Veer left on the trail and retrace your route to the junction where you first joined this trail. (After crossing the dirt road with the brown metal gate, stay right at an upcoming fork—the branches soon rejoin.) After reaching the junction where you first joined this trail, continue straight and then stay right at the next fork—the other branch soon merges on the left. Descend gently, curve left, and pass a faint path joining sharply from the left.

At the next fork, again stay right and after about 75 feet regain Westgate Road. Turn right, go about 100 feet, and then angle left onto a trail beside a big boulder (don't turn sharply left on the trail with two boulders). After about 75 feet you'll meet the Orange Trail at a junction. Turn left here and retrace your route to the parking area.

KEY AT-A-GLANCE INFORMATION

GENERAL

DISTANCE 1.8 miles

TYPE OF WALK Balloon

DIFFICULTY Easy

TIME TO WALK 1–2 hours

MAPS *Harwich*, USGS

SCENERY Forest, Herring River, reservoirs

EXPOSURE TO SUN Partial

TRAIL TRAFFIC Light

TRAIL SURFACE(S) Dirt

TRAILS OPEN All year

FEES/PASSES None

FACILITIES None

TRAIL USE

BICYCLES Allowed

DOGS Allowed on leash or under voice control

HUNTING Allowed in season

HEALTH STATS

NUMBER OF STEPS 4,050

ESTIMATED CALORIES BURNED 193

DIRECTIONS TO TRAILHEAD

From the intersection of Route 28 and Depot Road in West Harwich, take Depot Road north several hundred feet to a fork. Bear right on Bells Neck Road and go 1 mile to a very small dirt parking area, right. (If this area is full, you may park along the side of Bells Neck Road.)

Herring River

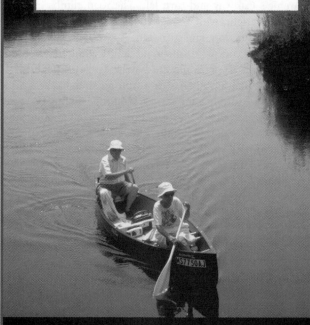

Calm waters of the Herring River are perfect for canoeing and kayaking.

WALK SUMMARY

This easy jaunt explores a conservation area bordering Harwich's Herring River. Along the way, you'll enjoy an overview of a vast cattail marsh and a look at a fish ladder designed to help migrating alewives reach their spawning grounds in West Reservoir. The route passes near some cranberry bogs, which are fun to visit except during midsummer, when black flies are rampant.

DESCRIPTION

Walk south from the parking area on Bells Neck Road, a wide dirt road on a narrow isthmus separating East and West reservoirs. This area is part of the Harwich Conservation Lands and is protected from development. West Reservoir, a flooded swamp, is a popular canoe and kayak put-in, giving

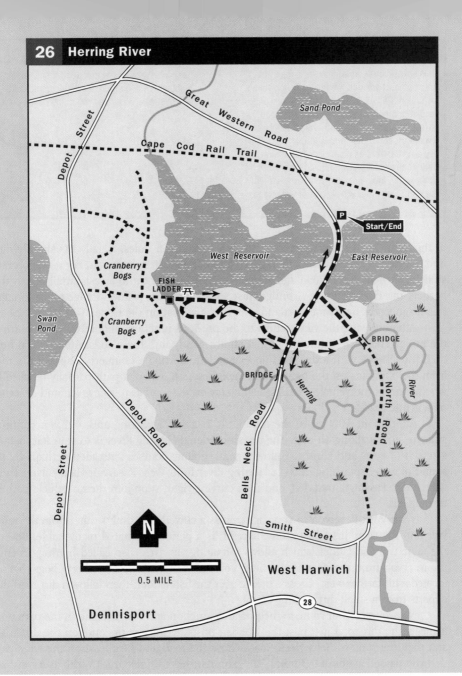

paddlers access to the Herring River, which traces a sinuous, mostly southward course to Nantucket Sound.

With an extensive marsh to the left and a hillside rising to the right, pass North Road on your left, which you will use later. Several more dirt roads depart

FLORA	FAUNA
This conservation area protects a forest of pitch pine, black oak, white oak, black cherry, red maple, bigtooth aspen, sumac, sassafras, and shadbush. Shrubs include arrowwood, sweet pepperbush, swamp azalea, highbush blueberry, scrub oak, and wild raisin. Poison ivy, Virginia creeper, greenbrier, bittersweet, and honeysuckle entwine beside the trail. Near water, look for cattails, alder, sweet gale, swamp rose, water willow, and pickerelweed.	Keep your eyes and ears open for such forest birds as black-capped chickadees, tufted titmice, gray catbirds, and mourning doves.

to the right, but keep walking straight. After about 0.3 miles, a trail cuts sharply right into the woods and a wide path angles left. You'll use these later, too. For now, continue straight on Bells Neck Road and soon emerge from forest into a vast cattail marsh that borders the Herring River. A bridge, just ahead, provides a fine vantage point to enjoy this magnificent freshwater wetland, one of the largest on the Cape.

After enjoying the view, return to the previous junction, about 100 yards north of the bridge and veer left on a trail that climbs gently into the woods. After several hundred feet, merge with a dirt road and angle left, skirting a cranberry bog. Soon a road from the bog joins on the right. At the next junction, where a path partially blocked by wooden posts (no vehicles) goes straight, stay on the road as it swings left and descends on a gentle grade.

After about 100 yards, the road ends at a small parking area and you continue straight, now walking on trail. The marsh-bordered Herring River is to your left, behind a screen of trees and shrubs. Follow a gently rolling course, serenaded perhaps by the sound of water splashing into the Herring River from West Reservoir via a culvert and a fish ladder. Passing a trail, left, and then curving right, soon join the no-vehicle path by turning left.

With West Reservoir to your right, cross a culvert that drains water from the reservoir into the river. Just ahead, on the right, is a perfectly situated picnic table. Beyond the table is a fish ladder, which allows migrating alewives, also called herring, to enter the reservoir from the river. (From here, you can explore several cranberry bogs that are located a bit farther west. Cross a bridge over the fish ladder; then follow a dirt road that departs from a small dirt parking area.)

Now retrace your route to the previous junction and stay straight on the path until it meets the dirt road just past the wooden posts. Retrace your route on the dirt road, and then the trail, to Bells Neck Road. Cross the road and head east on the wide path that you passed at about 0.3 miles. The path narrows to single-track width as it traverses level ground between a hillside on your left and a marsh on your right.

Just beyond two concrete barriers, you'll reach a loop at the end of North Road. To your right is a footbridge over the Herring River, another great vantage point for enjoying the scenery. Now follow North Road northwest to its junction with Bells Neck Road. From there, bear right and retrace your route to the parking area.

Kettle Pond Ramble

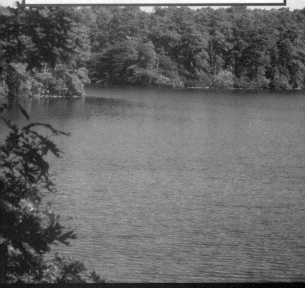

This undeveloped state park features classic Cape Cod kettle ponds.

WALK SUMMARY

This undeveloped state park is adjacent to busy Route 6, but as soon as you retreat into its forested realm, the traffic noise fades away and is replaced by bird song and the rustle of leaves. The route visits three kettle ponds surrounded by stately pines. Pick a dry spell to walk the trails and dirt roads here: they are muddy after it rains. Please respect all private property.

DESCRIPTION

To begin, visit lovely Hawksnest Pond by following a short trail north from the parking area to the pond's shore. If you're lucky, you may see one of the pond's namesake birds cruising overhead. After enjoying this pristine spot, return to the parking area and then walk a short distance to where the

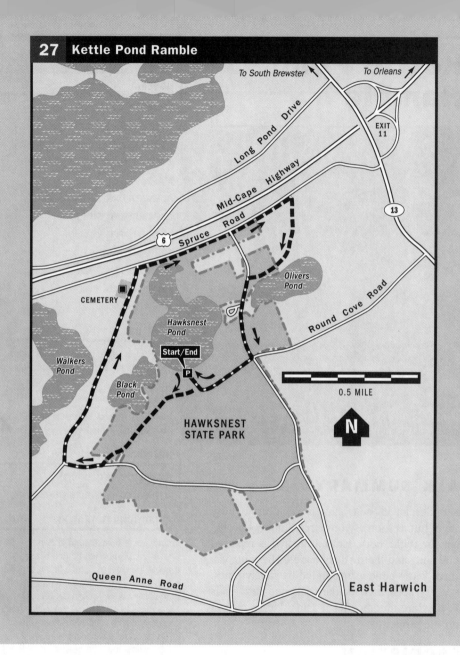

To South Brewster →
To Orleans ↗
Long Pond Drive
EXIT 11
Mid-Cape Highway
13
6 Spruce Road
Olivers Pond
CEMETERY
Round Cove Road
Hawksnest Pond
Walkers Pond
Start/End
P
Black Pond
0.5 MILE
N
HAWKSNEST STATE PARK
Queen Anne Road
East Harwich

dirt road dead-ends. Now climb southwest on a single-track trail that soon tops a rise and descends to near the southeast lobe of Black Pond.

After a trail departs right, merge with a narrow dirt road by angling right. Soon a trail goes left, but you continue straight to a junction with Nathan Walker Road, an unsigned dirt road. Here, in a clearing graced with a southern catalpa tree, you curve right. Go straight through the next junction, a four-way, and then stay right at a fork (private property to the left).

Where a dirt road goes left, you stay straight, skirting Black Pond, which is downhill right. At the next junction, a dirt road on the right offers access to Hawksnest Pond. Stay straight on Nathan Walker Road to its junction with paved Spruce Road, just past a historic cemetery with about a dozen headstones, some marking the graves of Revolutionary War veterans.

Now walk northeast on Spruce Road for 0.5 miles, staying left to face oncoming traffic. Just beyond where a roadside barrier on the right ends, find a blue fire hydrant and a junction. Turn right and enter forest on a wide trail that follows a rolling course to a trail fork. Stay right; the forks soon rejoin. After winding downhill and then uphill, reach another trail fork. Follow the right fork, climb moderately over a rise; then drop to meet the other branch of the fork, joining sharply from the left. Just ahead, a trail to Spruce Road departs right.

With Olivers Pond on your left, pass a trail, right, and then merge with a dirt road by veering left. Pass a small parking area and a trail climbing through the woods, both right, and then come to a dirt road signed private property. Your road curves left and climbs moderately through a dense woodland.

At a four-way junction, turn right on a dirt road. Descending gently, there are glimpses of Hawksnest Pond through a screen of trees and shrubs to your right. Next pass a wide path going left and then a trail to the pond on your right. Now climbing slightly, you soon close the loop at the parking area beside Hawksnest Pond.

GENERAL

DISTANCE 1.1 mile

TYPE OF WALK Balloon

DIFFICULTY Easy

TIME TO WALK 1–2 hours

MAPS *Morris Island Trail*, USFWS brochure with map; *Chatham*, USGS

SCENERY Beach, forest, islands, Nantucket Sound, salt marsh

EXPOSURE TO SUN Partial

TRAIL TRAFFIC Moderate

TRAIL SURFACE(S) Dirt, gravel, sand

TRAILS OPEN All year

FEES/PASSES None

FACILITIES Restrooms, water, visitor center

TRAIL USE

BICYCLES Trail not suitable for bicycles

DOGS Allowed on leash

HUNTING Not allowed from land; allowed in season from boat

HEALTH STATS

NUMBER OF STEPS 2,475

ESTIMATED CALORIES BURNED 118

DIRECTIONS TO TRAILHEAD

From the Route 28 rotary in Chatham, take Main Street southeast 0.8 miles to Shore Road. Turn right (still on Main Street) and go 0.5 miles south to a junction with Bridge Street and Morris Island Road. Go straight on Morris Island Road. After 0.3 miles, stay on Morris Island Road as it jogs right. Follow the road another 0.8 miles to Tisquantum Road. Angle left, drive 0.2 miles, turn left on Wikis Way, and go 0.1 mile to a paved parking area. The trailhead is on the east side of the parking area, beside an information board and just right of the restrooms.

Morris Island Trail

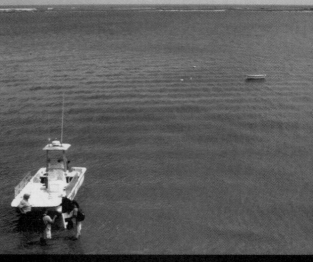

Morris Island Trail descends via steep steps to the beach, which is also used by boaters.

WALK SUMMARY

Most of Monomoy National Wildlife Refuge is accessible only by boat, but this short and easy stroll on Morris Island lets visitors see some of the same birds and plants that make North and South Monomoy islands—the bulk of the refuge—such special places. This walk is best done on a falling or rising tide; avoid high tide, as the route may be flooded. During summer, bring insect repellent.

Boldface numbers in the description below refer to numbered markers along the trail, which are keyed to text in "Morris Island Trail," a brochure available at the visitor center and online at **monomoy.fws.gov.** There are also interpretive panels along the trail, describing some of the area's wildlife and other features.

28   Morris Island Trail

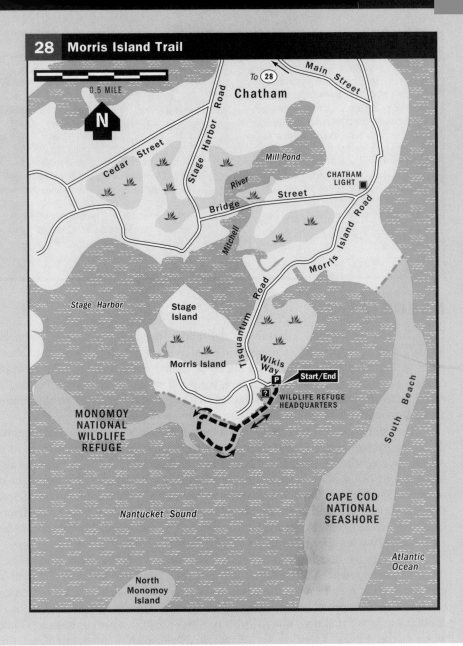

To visit North Monomoy Island or South Beach, there are two boat shuttles: Outermost Adventures, (508) 945-5858, **www.outermostharbor.com;** and Rip Ryder, (508) 945-5450, **www.monomoyislandferry.com.** Tours of North Monomoy Island and South Beach, as well as South Monomoy Island, are also available through Wellfleet Bay Wildlife Sanctuary, (508) 349-2615, **www.massaudubon.org/wellfleet.**

FLORA	FAUNA
For a small area, there is a great plant diversity here. In the forest, you'll find pitch pine, scrub oak, black oak, dwarf chestnut oak, black cherry, eastern red cedar, arrowwood, and shadbush. The understory includes low growers like bearberry, checkerberry, poverty grass, and huckleberry, and vines such as poison ivy, greenbrier, and honeysuckle. Summer and fall colors are provided by asters and goldenrods. Near the beach and the salt marsh, look for saltwater cordgrass, salt hay, cocklebur, sea lavender, marsh elder, sea blite, and glasswort.	Monomoy National Wildlife Refuge has been designated a World Bird Conservation Area by the American Bird Conservancy. The refuge is also a wilderness area and part of the Western Hemisphere Shorebird Reserve Network. So it's not surprising to find a welter of shorebirds here, including black-bellied plovers, semipalmated plovers, greater yellowlegs, short-billed dowitchers, red knots, ruddy turnstones, dunlin, semipalmated sandpipers, and sanderlings. Piping plovers, federally listed as a threatened species, nest on the refuge, as do endangered roseate terns. Also on view may be waterfowl and wading birds, along with songbirds in migration.

DESCRIPTION

From the trailhead, follow a boardwalk that curves right, passes marker **1** (songbird habitat), and enters a stand of shrubs and trees. A short dirt path leads left to a viewpoint with a couple of benches and marker **2** (island point lookout). The viewpoint offers a panorama of South Beach, a long barrier of sand and low dunes fronting the Atlantic Ocean. North Monomoy Island is southwest, and beyond it to the south is South Monomoy Island, whose lighthouse is visible with binoculars.

The landscape here is in flux, shaped by storms, winds, and tides. The Southway, the water passage between South Beach and the Monomoy Islands that leads to the Atlantic Ocean, silted in during the blizzard of 2005 and is impassable for most boats at low tide. In 1987, a storm broke through the barrier beach opposite Chatham Light and separated South Beach from Nauset Beach to the north. Now the south end of South Beach is curving west and may attach to South Monomoy, which would give predators a land route to the island. North and South Monomoy islands divided during a 1978 blizzard, about 20 years after being detached from Morris Island.

Return to the boardwalk, turn left, and stroll past a weather station and marker **3** (learning new vegetation). Where the boardwalk ends, bear right and walk about 40 feet on a sandy path; then turn left and descend via more boardwalk and steps, some steep, to a beach that disappears at high tide. Turn right and follow the sandy strand southwest about 0.1 mile to a trail sign, which directs you to the right to a path through low dunes, where marker **4** (wave action) awaits. As indicated by markers **5** and **6,** just ahead, these dunes provide enough protection for grasses, shrubs, and even small trees to take root and thrive, creating a stunted forest.

Now pass marker **7** (species diversity) and then turn left at a T-junction (not on the map), signed trail. Soon curve right to a fork, where another trail sign directs you left and up a slight rise that affords a view of Nantucket Sound. Nearby are marker **8** (salt-marsh ecosystems) and a small pond. (The right branch of the previous fork affords a close-up view of the pond.) Emerging from the trees and shrubs, you have an opportunity to study some common salt-marsh plants like sea lavender and sea rocket, as indicated by marker **9.**

The trail curves left and skirts the marsh, now running parallel to the beach. At about the 0.6-mile point, near marker **10** (shorebird habitat), you'll have an opportunity to scan the nearby beach for shorebirds. If the tide is low, the mudflats stretching west from North Monomoy Island may also be full of birds, but you'll need a spotting scope to identify them. The flats are also an important shellfishing area for the Town of Chatham.

Turn left at marker **10** and angle toward the beach. Merely a sandy track, the trail follows the high-tide line, which is marked by piles of seaweed, or wrack, and passes marker **11** (mudflats), which may be missing. Walking along the beach, soon close the loop at the junction where the trail crossed the dune. From here, continue straight and retrace your route to the parking area.

KEY AT-A-GLANCE INFORMATION

GENERAL

DISTANCE 1.1 mile

TYPE OF WALK Loop

DIFFICULTY Easy

TIME TO WALK 1 hour or less

MAPS *Orleans*, USGS

SCENERY Forest, Frostfish Cove, Little Pleasant Bay, The River

EXPOSURE TO SUN Partial

TRAIL TRAFFIC Moderate

TRAIL SURFACE(S) Dirt, wood chips

TRAILS OPEN All year

FEES/PASSES None

FACILITIES None

TRAIL USE

BICYCLES Allowed on dirt road; single-track trails not suitable for bicycles

DOGS Allowed on leash

HUNTING Not allowed

HEALTH STATS

NUMBER OF STEPS 2,475

ESTIMATED CALORIES BURNED 118

DIRECTIONS TO TRAILHEAD

From the Route 6 rotary at the Eastham-Orleans line, take Route 6A/28 south 0.5 miles to a fork, where Route 28, signed for Chatham and Falmouth, branches left. Bear left, go 0.4 miles to a traffic signal at Main Street, and turn left. Go 0.4 miles to Monument Road and turn right. Go 0.6 miles to Frost Fish Lane, turn left, and follow the unimproved, partially paved road for 0.2 miles to paved Keziah's Lane. Continue straight and go another 0.1 mile to a dirt-and-gravel parking area. There is an information board at the south end of the parking area with a sketch map of the named and color-coded trails. The trailhead is just behind the information board.

Kent's Point

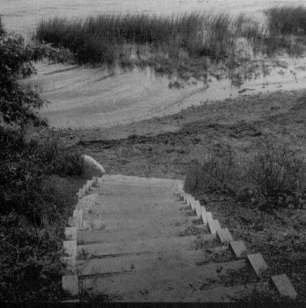

Steps lead down from the Brown Trail to the shore of The River, a waterway that connects to Little Pleasant Bay.

WALK SUMMARY

Don't let the small size fool you. Bordered by beautiful waterways, Kent's Point is a splendid swath of open space containing a surprising variety of both native and nonnative plants. This short but scenic loop rewards visitors with views of Frostfish Cove, The River, and Little Pleasant Bay. You can even take a short stroll on a sandy strand of beach. Before being acquired by the Town of Orleans as a conservation area, the land belonged to Charlotte A. Kent, who had a home here and also ran an artist colony on her property.

DESCRIPTION

To start, take the Cove Trail (Red), which angles southeast from the trailhead and soon passes a junction with the Blue Trail, right. Stay on the Cove Trail

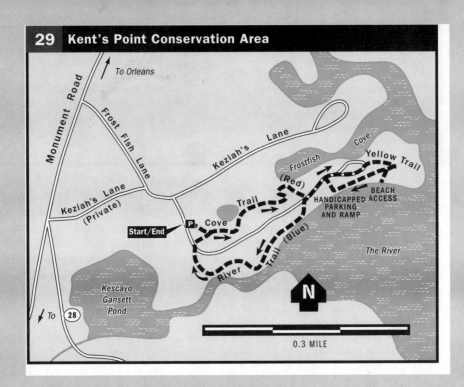

To Orleans

Monument Road

Frost Fish Lane

Keziah's Lane

Keziah's Lane (Private)

Keziah's Lane

Frostfish (Red) Trail

Cove

Yellow Trail

Cove

BEACH HANDICAPPED ACCESS PARKING AND RAMP

Start/End

P Cove

River Trail (Blue)

The River

Kescayo Gansett Pond

To 28

N

0.3 MILE

as it wanders through a shady forest, passes a rest bench, and climbs to a T-junction. Turn left and zigzag downhill, passing a short path, to your left, which leads to a rest bench overlooking the upper reaches of Frostfish Cove, fringed with salt marsh. Now climb gently to a T-junction with a dirt road and turn left.

After several hundred feet pass a handicapped-parking area, right, and a ramp leading to a viewpoint on The River, the name of a sinuous body of water that connects Meeting House Pond with Little Pleasant Bay. Continue on the dirt road, ignoring the paths that diverge left and right. Where a fork marks the start of a loop, you'll stay right. As the road begins to loop left, meet two trails—the Yellow Trail going straight, and another going right. Take the Yellow Trail, passing a clearing where Charlotte Kent's house once stood.

After the town of Orleans bought the property in 1988, all buildings were removed, but some of the plantings that mark this as a homesite—black locust, spruce, Norway maple, yew, and lilac—still remain. Nearing the end of Kent's point, pass the Brown Trail on your right and then come to a large bench that has a commanding view of The River and Little Pleasant Bay. After enjoying this restful spot, return to the previous junction. Veer left on the Brown Trail, which leads to a set of steps that provides beach access.

Beyond the steps, the trail continues to a T-junction. Here turn right, go 75 feet, regain the dirt road, and then turn left and retrace your route on the

FLORA	FAUNA
Despite its diminutive size—just under 28 acres—this open space has a fine variety of plants, including pitch pine, white pine, black oak, white oak, eastern red cedar, black cherry, American basswood, shadbush, bayberry, highbush blueberry, winterberry, and arrowwood.	Some of the common forest birds at home here are blue jays, tufted titmice, white-breasted nuthatches, downy woodpeckers, and black-capped chickadees.

dirt road. When you meet the Cove Trail, on the right, continue on the road another 50 feet or so. Then turn left on the River Trail (Blue), which winds between the water and the road. Several rest benches along the way invite you to sit and contemplate the wisdom of preserving parcels of open space such as this one.

In places, "windows" through the trees and shrubs afford views of the tidal channel that connects Kescayo Gansett Pond (aka Lonnie's Pond) to Little Pleasant Bay and provides a passage for alewives and blueback herring coming from the Atlantic Ocean to spawn in Pilgrim Lake. In places, paths cut right to join the dirt road: ignore these to stay on the described route.

At about the 1-mile point, just past a bench on your right, the trail surface changes to wood chips and makes a sharp right turn. Soon you'll meet the road, here dirt and gravel, at a T-junction. Turn left, go about 100 feet, and then veer right on a trail into the woods. After closing the loop at the Cove Trail, turn left and retrace your route to the parking area.

Bayside Stroll

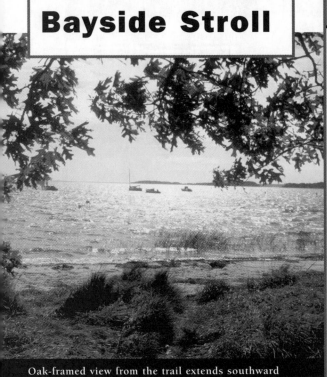

Oak-framed view from the trail extends southward across Little Pleasant Bay.

KEY AT-A-GLANCE INFORMATION

GENERAL

DISTANCE 0.4 miles

TYPE OF WALK Balloon

DIFFICULTY Easy

TIME TO WALK 30 minutes

MAPS *Orleans*, USGS

SCENERY Forest, Little Pleasant Bay, Paw Wah Pond

EXPOSURE TO SUN None

TRAIL TRAFFIC Light

TRAIL SURFACE(S) Dirt

TRAILS OPEN All year

FEES/PASSES None

FACILITIES None

TRAIL USE

BICYCLES Trails not suitable for bicycles

DOGS Allowed on leash

HUNTING Not allowed

HEALTH STATS

NUMBER OF STEPS 900

ESTIMATED CALORIES BURNED 43

DIRECTIONS TO TRAILHEAD

From the Route 6 rotary at the Eastham-Orleans line, take Route 6A/28 south 0.5 miles to a fork where Route 28, signed for Chatham and Falmouth, branches left. Bear left on Route 28, go 2.5 miles to Namequoit Road, and turn left. Go 1.1 mile to a dirt parking area, right. The trailhead is on the south-east corner of the parking area.

WALK SUMMARY

"Short and sweet" describes this lovely loop along a forested track beside Little Pleasant Bay. Forest, a fringe of salt march, and a sandy strand of Pleasant Bay beach combine to produce a scenic stroll that's perfect to walk with kids, or with coworkers on your lunch hour.

DESCRIPTION

From the trailhead, walk into a wooded area and past a junction with the return leg of the loop, which joins from the right. On a wide path carpeted with pine needles, curve right and pass a rest bench where the breeze from Pleasant Bay may be rustling the leaves above. Now with a bench on the right, the trail bends left and descends to a four-way junction.

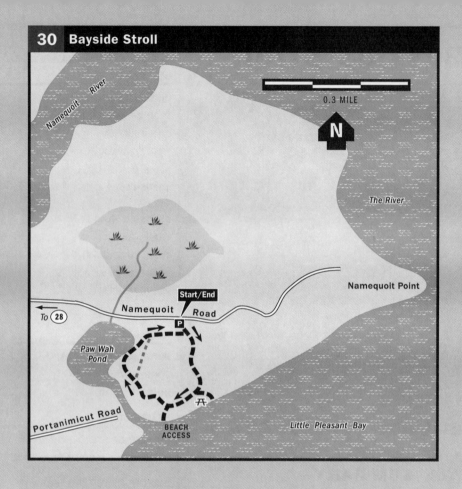

From here a short trail goes straight to a picnic table. Turn left and follow a narrow, winding path to a beach on Little Pleasant Bay. The view extends east to lands of Cape Cod National Seashore and south to Sipson and Strong islands in Pleasant Bay. A nearby town landing may have a fine collection of watercraft moored close to shore. Mats of dried eelgrass, a saltwater plant whose presence indicates a healthy ecosystem, may be strewn on the beach.

Now return to the previous junction, located beside the picnic table. Continue straight, go several hundred feet to a T-junction, and turn left. In about 100 feet, reach a well-placed bench overlooking Little Pleasant Bay. A set of steps leads from the bench to the beach, where there is an interpretive panel that lists common salt-marsh plants and animals. Return to the previous junction, go straight, and then follow the path on a serpentine course through an impressive pine forest with tall and stout trees.

FLORA

Underfoot are two common types of pine needles: green, stiff, in bundles of three (pitch pine); and blue-green, soft, in bundles of five (white pine). Black oak, white oak, black cherry, Virginia creeper, poison ivy, and greenbrier are at home in the forest. Beside the beach, look for such salt-marsh plants as saltwater cordgrass and salt hay.

FAUNA

Blue jays, black-capped chickadees, northern harriers, and great blue herons are some of the birds you may spot. Harder to see, because they are nocturnal, are mammals such as skunks, foxes, and raccoons—look for their tracks in wet sand or mud.

Where a trail branches left, follow it to a bench with a peekaboo view through the trees of Paw Wah Pond, which opens to Little Pleasant Bay. Continue past the bench, curve right, and meet the main trail at a T-junction. Here turn left and soon close the loop just south of the trailhead. Turn left and retrace your route to the parking area.

Cape Cod: Outer Cape

GENERAL

DISTANCE 4.3 miles

TYPE OF WALK Balloon

DIFFICULTY Moderate

TIME TO WALK 2–3 hours

MAPS *The Nauset Marsh Trail,* CCNS brochure with map; *Cape Cod National Seashore,* National Geographic Maps; *Orleans,* USGS

SCENERY Atlantic Ocean, forest, Nauset Marsh, Salt Pond

EXPOSURE TO SUN Partial

TRAIL TRAFFIC Heavy

TRAIL SURFACE(S) Dirt, gravel, pavement

TRAILS OPEN All year

FEES/PASSES None

FACILITIES Restrooms, water, visitor center, phone

TRAIL USE

BICYCLES Not allowed

DOGS Not allowed

HUNTING Not allowed

HEALTH STATS

NUMBER OF STEPS 9,675

ESTIMATED CALORIES BURNED 461

DIRECTIONS TO TRAILHEAD

From the southernmost intersection of Route 6 and Nauset Road in Eastham, marked by a traffic signal and a sign for Cape Cod National Seashore's Salt Pond visitor center, take Nauset Road northeast a few hundred feet; then turn right into a large paved parking area. The Salt Pond visitor center is adjacent to the parking area. The trailhead for the Nauset Marsh and Buttonbush trails is on the southwest corner of the parking area, between the visitor center and the restrooms.

Nauset Marsh Trail and Coast Guard Beach

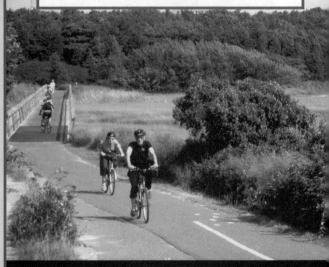

A paved bicycle trail connects Salt Pond visitor center and Coast Guard Beach parking area.

WALK SUMMARY

Don't miss this scenic stroll beside Nauset Marsh, one of the Cape's natural wonders and setting for two classics of nature writing—*The Outermost House,* by Henry Beston, and *The House on Nauset Marsh,* by Wyman Richardson. The Richardson house still stands, but Beston's cabin, which was nestled in the dunes on Coast Guard Beach, was last seen floating out to sea during the blizzard of 1978. The mostly level trail winds through forest and beside the marsh, giving you the chance to study some of the area's plants and wildlife. Trailside markers identify some common trees and shrubs.

DESCRIPTION

From the trailhead, follow a paved path downhill, just right of an amphitheater, passing a box for trail

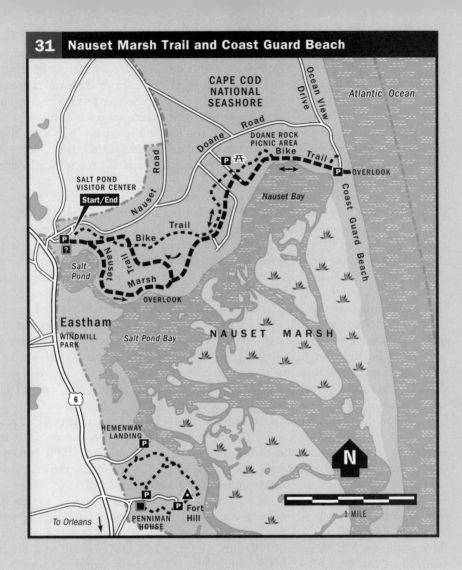

brochures. Now on a dirt-and-gravel trail, soon reach Salt Pond, a circular kettle pond connected to Salt Pond Bay in Nauset Marsh by a narrow channel. From here, bear left and follow a sandy trail and an elevated boardwalk that skirt the pond's north shore. A boat landing, visible to the right, is a favorite with canoers and kayakers heading to the marsh, one of the Cape's best paddling destinations. The trail bends left and follows the narrow channel, which may have a swift tidal current.

When you reach a fork, stay right unless the tide is high and the trail flooded; then stay left. The fork's branches soon rejoin near a rest bench. Salt Pond Bay, part of the Nauset Marsh, is just ahead. The marsh consists of various bays, channels, and islands—all protected from the Atlantic Ocean by a barrier beach and low dunes. The marsh floods at high tide and parts of it nearly empty at low.

Now cross a dike with a bridge over a little creek that feeds a salt marsh, which is on the left. Stroll a few paces, turning left and then right, to enter a forest of eastern red cedar and climb moderately on widely spaced dirt steps reinforced with logs. The curvy climb leads to a level stretch through a serene forest. When you reach a clearing, a vantage point with rest benches affords the first real look at the expanse of Nauset Marsh, extending south to Fort Hill in Eastham and southeast to Nauset Heights in Orleans. You may even be able to see the break in the barrier beach, which allows cold North Atlantic water to fill the marsh.

Now descend via dirt steps and enjoy a level walk beside a salt marsh. Soon reach a junction where the Nauset Marsh Trail turns left and a trail to the Doane Memorial and Coast Guard Beach goes right. (To shorten the walk, turn left and walk 0.7 miles to the visitor center.) Turn right toward Doane Memorial and follow a dirt trail that wanders through alternating open and wooded areas on a gently rolling course, passing a partially overgrown pond, which is right. At about the 1-mile point, reach a four-way junction with a dirt-and-gravel road, which you cross.

The route now rises steadily on a gentle grade, soon entering a mixed forest. A short, slalom descent leads to a level, meandering course for about 0.3 miles to a junction. Here a short trail goes straight to the bicycle trail (paved), but you curve right and walk parallel to the paved trail. Topping a low rise, drop to meet a paved road, which you cross. Soon reach a T-junction with a paved path, where you turn right. (To visit Doane Rock, a large glacial boulder, turn left. Near the rock are a parking area, picnic tables, and a seasonal restroom.)

Follow the paved path for about 150 feet. Just before the path merges with a paved road, there is an interpretive panel on the right, which tells the early history of this area, settled in 1644 by seven families from Plymouth. Deacon John Doane (1590–1685) was one of this group. The other family names were Bangs, Cook, Higgins, Prence, Smalley, and Snow. These names still resonate today as you wander the Cape.

Now go straight on the paved road to a four-way junction. About 40 feet ahead is a memorial, erected in 1869 by Doane's descendants, which marks the Doane homesite. Turn left (northeast) at the four-way junction and follow a paved path, passing a rest bench, which is left. After about 100 yards, turn right and walk downhill on a dirt trail, signed for Coast Guard Beach. (The path going straight here is another route to Doane Rock.) Dirt steps lead downhill to the edge of a salt marsh, where the trail curves left.

The view from here takes in Nauset Bay, a large shallow area at the northeast corner of Nauset Marsh. An old Coast Guard Station that stands on a bluff overlooking Nauset Bay now serves as an environmental education center.

Just shy of 2 miles, after a short stretch of boardwalk and more dirt trail, meet the bicycle trail at a T-junction. Here turn right on the paved trail, staying to its right side. Soon step onto a much longer boardwalk that carries you across an expanse of marsh and a narrow channel. At the east end of the boardwalk, the bike trail curves left, but angle slightly right on a dirt trail that climbs through an old pear orchard mixed with eastern red cedar.

After emerging at the parking area for Coast Guard Beach, walk northeast, diagonally across the parking area, and then follow a paved path east between the education center and restrooms (seasonal) to an overlook above Coast Guard Beach and the Atlantic Ocean. Interpretive panels here describe some of the human and natural history that make this part of the Cape so special. When ready to resume the walk, retrace your route to the junction with the Nauset Marsh Trail, at about 3.6 miles. Here, angle right and follow a sign for the visitor center. Climb on widely spaced dirt steps and then follow a rolling course, descending via a single switchback and traversing near a shrub-bordered pond.

Now climb on widely spaced dirt steps away from the pond. When you meet the bike trail at a four-way junction, cross it and continue on the Nauset Marsh Trail. Nauset Road is immediately right, behind a screen of vegetation. After crossing a paved driveway, continue following the trail, with the bike trail still on your left. Soon cross the bike trail, go about 200 feet, and turn left on the Buttonbush Trail (here part of the Nauset Marsh Trail), a wide dirt-and-gravel loop designed to highlight nonvisual features. The trail has a guide rope and text panels in Braille and large lettering. Soon the other end of the Buttonbush Trail joins sharply from the right. Go about 25 feet to a T-junction with a paved path. The amphitheater is left and the parking area is right.

GENERAL

DISTANCE 1.5 miles

TYPE OF WALK Loop

DIFFICULTY Moderate

TIME TO WALK 1–2 hours

MAPS *Fort Hill Trail,* CCNS brochure with map; *Orleans,* USGS

SCENERY Red maple swamp, Nauset Marsh, historic house

EXPOSURE TO SUN Partial

TRAIL TRAFFIC Heavy

TRAIL SURFACE(S) Boardwalk, dirt, pavement

TRAILS OPEN All year

FEES/PASSES None

FACILITIES Restroom (seasonal), located partway around loop

TRAIL USE

BICYCLES Not allowed

DOGS Not allowed

HUNTING Not allowed

HEALTH STATS

NUMBER OF STEPS 3,375

ESTIMATED CALORIES BURNED 161

DIRECTIONS TO TRAILHEAD

From Route 6 northbound in Eastham, go 1.4 miles northeast of the Eastham–Orleans rotary and angle right on Governor Prence Road, signed for the Fort Hill Area. Go 0.2 miles, turn right on Fort Hill Road, and go 0.1 mile to a small parking area, left.

From Route 6 southbound in Eastham, go 1.3 miles south of the Salt Pond visitor center and turn left on Governor Prence Road, marked by a flashing yellow light and signed for the Fort Hill Area. Go 0.1 mile, to where Governor Prence Road turns right and Fort Hill Road goes straight. Take Fort Hill Road 0.1 mile to a small parking area on your left.

Red Maple Swamp and Fort Hill

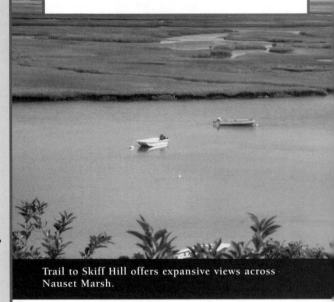

Trail to Skiff Hill offers expansive views across Nauset Marsh.

WALK SUMMARY

This rewarding loop combines two terrific trails— one that explores the Red Maple Swamp, the other that circles Fort Hill. Along the way, you'll encounter a number of different habitats—kettle-hole swamp, forest, open fields, salt marsh—and with them a plethora of plants and birds. Part of the route overlooks Nauset Marsh, which inspired two classics of nature writing, Henry Beston's *Outmost House,* and Wyman Richardson's *The House on Nauset Marsh.* On a walk that visits a swamp and a marsh, don't be surprised to encounter mosquitoes and other biting insects: cover up and bring repellent.

DESCRIPTION

The trailhead is on the northeast corner of the parking area, beside a CCNS map and a box for trail

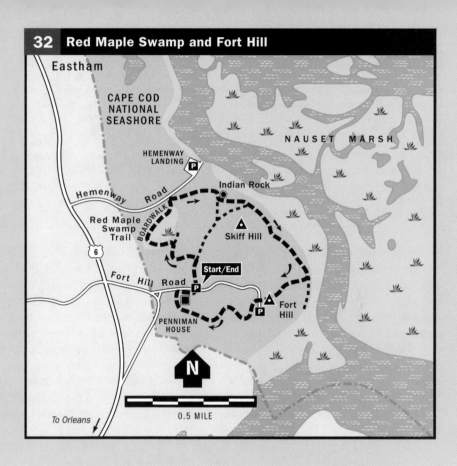

Eastham

CAPE COD
NATIONAL
SEASHORE

NAUSET MARSH

HEMENWAY
LANDING

Hemenway Road

Indian Rock

Red Maple
Swamp
Trail

BOARDWALK

Skiff Hill

6

Fort Hill Road

Start/End

Fort
Hill

PENNIMAN
HOUSE

N

0.5 MILE

To Orleans

brochures (which may be empty). Follow the Fort Hill Trail, which heads north-east between a wooded area, left, and an open field, right. After about 100 yards, reach a junction, where you turn left on the Red Maple Swamp Trail. The swamp lies in the bottom of a glacial kettle hole, and as you descend, a dense forest sur-rounds you. Where the trail levels, look for the swamp's namesake trees, which have lobed leaves with red stems. In autumn, the leaves turn a rusty red. Red maples can grow to 75 feet or more, but they have shallow roots, which makes them susceptible to toppling.

Gaining a boardwalk, follow a curvy course through the swamp with rest benches along the way. At a wide fork, angle left and continue to follow the boardwalk as it zigs, zags, and wanders across the kettle hole's bottom. Like the Cape's many ponds, this kettle hole was formed by a chunk of ice left behind by a glacier. Once the kettle hole was steep-walled, but erosion has lessened the angle of the surrounding hillsides.

Some of the old maples here have elaborately twisted trunks, which make them perfect subjects for photographs. In places, the forest canopy thins, and

FLORA	FAUNA
In the Red Maple Swamp are, of course, red maples, but also white oak, tupelo, arrow-wood, sweet pepperbush, highbush blueberry, winterberry, ferns, poison ivy, Virginia creeper, berry and grape vines, and briars. Elsewhere on the walk, look for eastern red cedar, black oak, black cherry, and bayberry. In season, the open fields are full of wildflowers, including goldenrods, asters, chicory, yarrow, and Queen Anne's lace. There is even a stand of lupine, which blooms in late spring and early summer. Fruit trees attest to the area's farming past.	Fort Hill, with its open fields bordered by forest, is perfect for songbirds. Look (and listen) for American goldfinches, black-capped chickadees, swallows, gray catbirds, eastern kingbirds, red-winged blackbirds, and northern bobwhites. Nauset Marsh, one of the Cape's premier bird-watching spots, hosts herons, egrets, ducks, gulls, terns, shorebirds, and birds of prey.

the added sunlight stimulates a riot of vegetation, which forms impenetrable thickets just beside the boardwalk. Eventually the boardwalk forks left to Hemenway Road, but you go straight on a path that climbs via log steps to a paved path. Turn right, passing restrooms (seasonal) on your left, and climb to an overlook of Nauset Marsh, left. There are rest benches here, and the view extends across the marsh to the Atlantic Ocean. An old Coast Guard station, now an environmental education center, stands on a bluff to the northeast.

Continue uphill for several hundred feet to Skiff Hill and Sharpening Rock, which was used by Native Americans to grind implements of stone and animal bones. Look for a shelter and several interpretive panels. One shows a map, still fairly accurate, from Samuel de Champlain's 1605 exploration of the area. Just south of the shelter are two trails, one going straight (south), the other left (southeast). To shorten the walk, take the south trail 0.3 miles to the parking area. Otherwise, veer left on the southeast trail.

Soon a trail departs left but rejoins after several hundred feet. Next, a short connector cuts right to meet the Fort Hill Trail. Stay left, walk about 100 feet, and merge with the Fort Hill Trail by angling left. After 100 yards, the trail bends left to skirt the remains of a stone wall, one of several that traverse the large open field to your right. Part of Fort Hill was once owned by the Reverend Samuel Treat (1648–1717), Eastham's first resident minister, and the land has a long history of agricultural use.

After reaching a large glacial boulder and a junction, a short trail goes straight to an overlook of Nauset Marsh, and the Fort Hill Trail goes right. Turn right and climb to a parking area atop Fort Hill. There is a magnificent view from here southeast across Nauset Marsh. Walk across the parking area and descend along a mowed path southwest about 100 yards to forest. Now on a dirt trail, wander at little more than 0.1 mile through woods to the Penniman House, which you skirt on its south and west sides. Captain Edward Penniman, who at age 29 became master of his own whaling ship, built the house in 1868.

Rock steps lead you from the lawn of the house down to Fort Hill Road, where you turn right. Soon pass the jawbones of a whale, which many photographers have used to frame the house. Go another 100 feet or so, and cross Fort Hill Road to the parking area.

Atlantic White Cedar Swamp Trail

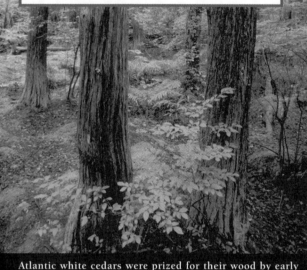

Atlantic white cedars were prized for their wood by early settlers, who used them for everything from fence posts to organ pipes.

KEY AT-A-GLANCE INFORMATION

GENERAL

DISTANCE 1.2 miles

TYPE OF WALK Loop

DIFFICULTY Easy

TIME TO WALK 1 hour or less

MAPS *Atlantic White Cedar Swamp Trail*, CCNS brochure with map; *Wellfleet*, USGS

SCENERY White cedar swamp

EXPOSURE TO SUN Partial

TRAIL TRAFFIC Moderate

TRAIL SURFACE(S) Dirt, sand

TRAILS OPEN All year

FEES/PASSES None

FACILITIES Restrooms, water (both seasonal), picnic table

TRAIL USE

BICYCLES Not allowed

DOGS Not allowed

HUNTING Not allowed

HEALTH STATS

NUMBER OF STEPS 2,700

ESTIMATED CALORIES BURNED 129

DIRECTIONS TO TRAILHEAD

From Route 6 in South Wellfleet, at a traffic signal signed for the Marconi Station Area, take Marconi Beach Road east 0.1 mile; then turn left on Marconi Station Road, following signs for the Marconi Station Site. Go another 1 mile to a loop parking area. The trailhead is on the west side of the parking area, near its entrance. *Note:* There is no beach access here.

WALK SUMMARY

This mostly shaded loop, great on a hot day, explores one of the Cape's few remaining stands of Atlantic white cedar, located on the former site of Camp Wellfleet, a U.S. Army base. Trailside markers identify many of the common plants, and you'll probably get to see and hear some forest birds as well. The swamp usually has standing water, so bring mosquito repellent.

The Marconi Station Site, located just across the parking area from the trailhead, is well worth a visit. When Morse-code messages between President Theodore Roosevelt and England's King Edward VII were exchanged from here on January 18, 1903, the age of two-way wireless communication began.

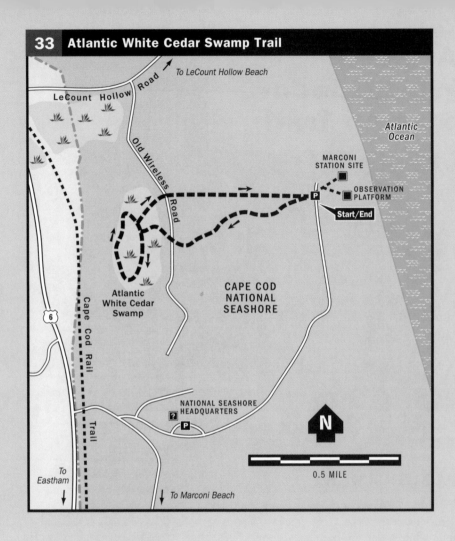

To LeCount Hollow Beach

LeCount Hollow Road

Old Wireless Road

Atlantic
Ocean

MARCONI
STATION SITE

OBSERVATION
PLATFORM

Start/End

Atlantic
White Cedar
Swamp

CAPE COD
NATIONAL
SEASHORE

Cape Cod Rail

6

Trail

NATIONAL SEASHORE
HEADQUARTERS

P

N

To
Eastham

To Marconi Beach

0.5 MILE

DESCRIPTION

Begin the walk along a sandy trail lined with logs, passing a rest bench—
on your left—to a fork. Take the left fork, passing a box for trail brochures, and
follow an avenue of wind-stunted pitch pines and scrub oaks. The route winds
generally westward on a level course, then descends via widely spaced dirt
steps. Another level stretch wanders through a classic pine–oak forest. After an
up and a down, the trail curves right and comes to the first area of standing
water (except during dry periods).

Soon cross a dirt road and find the continuation of the trail. Just ahead is a
boardwalk that leads you into a realm of Atlantic white cedars. These magnificent

evergreens, which can grow to 90 feet tall, were prized for their wood by the early settlers, who used them for everything from fence posts to roof rafters to organ pipes. Gunpowder for the Revolutionary War came from white-cedar charcoal. Logged heavily, only a few stands like the one here remain on the Cape.

Passing a rest bench, left, you come to a fork in the boardwalk. Stay left and traverse the swamp, which sits in the bottom of a kettle hole. Most of the ponds on the Cape are kettle holes, so picture this as a pond with very little water. The boardwalk makes a long, curvy course through the swamp, eventually swinging 180 degrees to the right and coming to a T-junction. The right-hand branch leads to several rest benches and then to the fork you passed earlier.

Turn left at the T-junction and soon regain a sandy trail, which climbs gently through a pine–oak forest. Now you reach a potentially confusing junction with several dirt roads. Continue straight and merge with Old Wireless Road by angling slightly right. This dirt road dates from around 1903, when Marconi's station was active. Passing a rest bench, left, ascend in the open and close the loop at the junction near the trail-brochure box. From there, retrace your route to the parking area.

KEY AT-A-GLANCE INFORMATION

GENERAL

DISTANCE 7.2 miles

TYPE OF WALK Out-and-back

DIFFICULTY Difficult

TIME TO WALK 3–5 hours

MAPS *Great Island Trail,* CCNS brochure with map; *Wellfleet,* USGS

SCENERY Beach, forest, salt marsh

EXPOSURE TO SUN Partial

TRAIL TRAFFIC Moderate

TRAIL SURFACE(S) Dirt, sand

TRAILS OPEN All year

FEES/PASSES None

FACILITIES Toilets (seasonal), picnic areas

TRAIL USE

BICYCLES Not allowed on upland parts of the route, including the interior of Great Island and Great Beach Hill

DOGS Not allowed on upland parts of the route, including the interior of Great Island and Great Beach Hill

HUNTING Not allowed

HEALTH STATS

NUMBER OF STEPS 16,200

ESTIMATED CALORIES BURNED 771

DIRECTIONS TO TRAILHEAD

From Route 6 northbound in Wellfleet, turn left on Main Street at the first Wellfleet exit, marked by traffic signal and a sign for Wellfleet center and harbor. Go 0.3 miles and turn left onto East Commercial Street, which soon becomes Commercial Street. Go 0.7 miles to the Wellfleet marina. Follow the road as it bends right and becomes Kendrick Avenue. Go 0.7 miles to an intersection with Chequessett Neck Road. Bear left and follow Chequessett Neck Road 1.7 miles to Griffin Island Road. Bear left; after about 200 feet turn left into a large parking area marked with a brown National Seashore sign for Great Island. *Note:* For directions from Route 6 southbound, see end of Description.

Great Island Trail

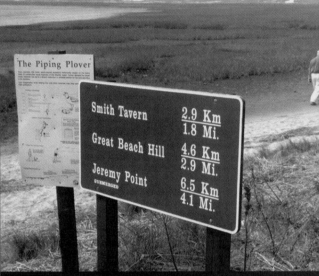

Great Island Trail is one of the Cape's premier walks, visiting salt marsh, beach, and forest.

WALK SUMMARY

This hike, one of the best on Cape Cod, explores the dunes, salt marshes, and upland forests on Griffin Island, Great Island, and Great Beach Hill, all part of Cape Cod National Seashore. Great Island, Great Beach Hill, and a protruding sand spit called Jeremy Point form the boundary between Wellfleet Harbor and Cape Cod Bay. The area contains one of the longest continuous expanses of undeveloped beach on the Cape, and abounds in native plants and birds. Save this walk for a cool day, bring plenty of water, and be prepared to slog through stretches of soft sand and piles of matted marsh grass. *Note:* Parts of the route may be flooded by high tides; parts of Jeremy Point are submerged at high tide.

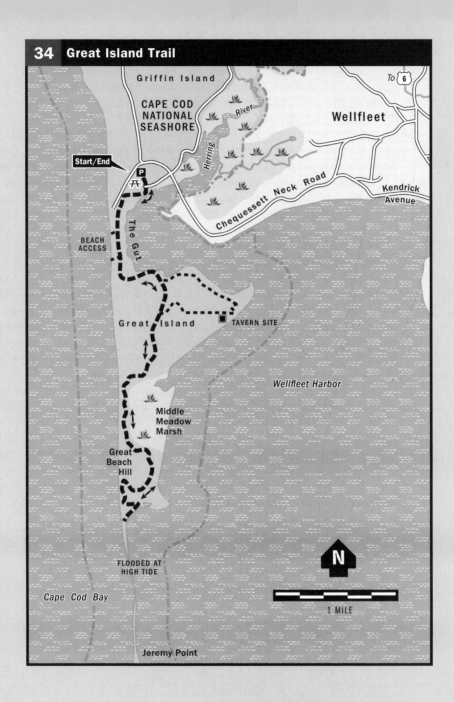

Griffin Island

CAPE COD NATIONAL SEASHORE

Herring River

Wellfleet

To 6

Start/End

P

BEACH ACCESS

The Gut

Chequessett Neck Road

Kendrick Avenue

Great Island

TAVERN SITE

Wellfleet Harbor

Middle Meadow Marsh

Great Beach Hill

N

FLOODED AT HIGH TIDE

Cape Cod Bay

1 MILE

Jeremy Point

DESCRIPTION

Go east from the trailhead on a broad gravel path. Several hundred feet from the trailhead, on the right, are a memorial to a Wampanoag woman and an interpretive panel describing the Great Island tavern site, a fabled retreat for local shore whalers in search of whiskey and women. In 1970, archaeologists digging on Great Island found thousands of artifacts and the foundation of a building, which they say was in use from around 1690 to 1740. The artifacts were removed and there are no visible remains of the site today.

The path soon heads downhill toward a salt marsh, ending with a set of steps leading to a T-junction with a wide, sandy path. This marsh is where the meandering Herring River widens, swings southeast, and empties into Wellfleet Harbor. As you take the last couple of steps downhill, look out across the marsh. As you face south, Wellfleet Harbor is on your left, and Cape Cod Bay is beyond the dunes to your right. Great Island is one of a chain of former islands in Wellfleet that are connected by low-lying strips of sand called tombolos. From north to south these "islands" are Bound Brook, Merrick, Griffin and Great islands, and Great Beach Hill.

This marsh is a good place to observe the dramatic effect of the tides. Because Wellfleet Harbor is shallow, the area flooded at high tide is much greater than the area covered at low water. The high-tide line separates two very different plant communities—salt marsh and sand dune. If it is low tide, you'll notice mud flats and exposed marsh plants, and perhaps feeding shorebirds. If it is high tide, this area could be flooded up to, and sometimes over, the path.

At the T-junction, turn right on the dirt path. After about 300 yards, the path curves left and comes to a boardwalk and the start of a split-rail fence, right. Notice the large meadow of salt hay, left. Over the course of several centuries, meadows of salt hay were used as pastures and harvested to provide fodder for livestock. This area, where a narrow tombolo connects Griffin and Great islands, is known locally as The Gut. At one time, the Herring River emptied into Cape Cod Bay through here. Soon you'll reach the first of two access paths, on your right, that lead uphill and through the dunes to the beach. You can get a fine view of Cape Cod Bay by climbing either path. From late spring

To visit the Great Island tavern site, bear left along the edge of the marsh, round a point, and then continue along a sandy beach in a lovely cove. About 0.6 miles from the previous junction, a sign indicates a trail that climbs into low dunes. Further signs and interpretive panels with photographs of the archeological dig lead the way to the tavern site, which is merely a depression in the ground where archaeologists uncovered and removed artifacts. Just ahead of the site, a short path branches left to a beautiful overlook with a view of Wellfleet Harbor. Beyond the site, the trail heads west and rejoins the main trail about 0.2 miles south from where the two trails diverged.
To shorten the walk, turn right, go about 0.2 miles, and then bear left and retrace your route to the parking area.

FLORA	FAUNA
A variety of habitats ensures a variety of plants. At higher elevations, pitch pines and black oaks dominate, with an occasional black cherry, white poplar, and eastern red cedar. Shrubs here include bayberry, beach plum, scrub oak, and salt-spray rose, with a ground cover of bearberry, poison ivy, and Virginia creeper. Pink lady's slippers and starflower grow beneath the pines.	Beginning in July, shorebirds returning from their northern breeding grounds begin to congregate in the marshes and along the beaches of Cape Cod, joining local nesters and year-round residents. A visit to Jeremy Point in season is likely to yield American oystercatchers, whimbrels, semipalmated plovers, piping plovers, greater yellowlegs, ruddy turnstones, sanderlings, and semipalmated sandpipers. Gulls and terns may be present in large flocks.
The route's three salt marshes and their borders contain saltwater cordgrass, salt hay, sea lavender, glasswort, sea blite, and orach. The dunes host American beach grass, seaside goldenrod, bouncing bet, cocklebur, dusty miller, wormwood, poverty grass, and beach pea.	In moist sand and mud beside the marsh, you may notice fiddler crabs and their tiny burrows. Watch them darting back and forth, the males holding their one large claw aloft. As you approach, the crabs scuttle into their holes. Fiddler crabs are great excavators, leaving little mounds of balled sediment as they improve their holes and tunnels. These tiny crabs provide an important food source for migrating shorebirds, especially whimbrels.

through midsummer, these paths are closed at high tide to protect nesting shorebirds. (Elsewhere, unofficial trails cut across the dunes to the Bay—please do not use these.)

At the southwest corner of the marsh, your route bends left and heads toward Wellfleet Harbor. A little past the 1-mile point is a signed junction. Here the main trail angles right, and a trail to the Great Island tavern site, where nothing but a shallow depression remains, goes left (see sidebar on previous page).

Now bear right and enter a mostly pine forest. The trail soon crests a low hill and then begins a gentle descent. Here a few oaks are gaining a foothold in a shady forest dominated mostly by pitch pines. The pines were planted in the 1830s to control erosion after the old-growth hardwoods had been cut. Eventually, the pines will die and the oaks and other hardwoods will prevail—this process is called succession.

Now you meet the trail from the tavern site, which joins on the left. About 300 yards ahead is a monument commemorating Priscilla Alden Bartlett, a descendant of Mayflower passenger and Massachusetts governor William Bradford. Bartlett and her husband, Alexander I. Henderson, were the last private owners of Great Island.

This is such a woodsy and secluded area that it is easy to forget you are walking on a narrow strip of land, with water on either side. The route rises moderately and then descends toward a second salt marsh, called Middle Meadow Marsh. Here the sound of waves and the refreshing coastal breeze mean that water is near. The route now curves right and then bends left to follow the west edge of the marsh, beside the tombolo connecting Great Island and Great Beach Hill. Cape Cod Bay is across the low dunes to the west.

As you reach the southwest corner of the marsh, the route begins to climb a dune where a sign announces GREAT BEACH HILL, and a moderate trudge over soft sand puts you once more in forest. Notice how short the pine trees have become as you gain elevation and leave the shelter of the mainland behind. This gives you some idea of the power of winter storms that roar through here, with winds generally out of the northeast.

The route descends gently to a third salt marsh. From here, the land dwindles to a narrow spit, ending in the far distance at Jeremy Point. This can be a windy area, with only low dunes for shelter. Beyond Jeremy Point is Billingsgate Island, once the site of a prosperous town but now, after centuries of erosion, a sandy, rock-strewn shoal exposed only at low tide.

The route curves right, skirts the edge of the third marsh, and soon comes to the last few trees—beyond are only dune plants and marsh vegetation. A sign that says you've come 2.9 miles marks a junction. Here a sandy path climbs over a low dune to Cape Cod Bay. Your route, however, turns sharply left to trace the west edge of the marsh. As the dunes get lower and lower, Cape Cod Bay comes into view to the west, and you can see both the Bay and Wellfleet Harbor simultaneously.

A sandy path through a gully branches to the right but soon rejoins. Follow the marsh edge as it curves left, toward Wellfleet Harbor. When you reach a sandy beach, bear right another 0.1 mile or so, to where an access path cuts right, through the dune, to Cape Cod Bay. Ahead there is one more low dune with beach grass, roped off in season to protect nesting shorebirds, and then nothing but beach and mudflats. (Use caution when venturing farther if the tide is rising.)

On a clear day views stretch northwest across Cape Cod Bay to the Pilgrim Monument in Provincetown. Across Wellfleet Harbor to the east are the highlands of Indian Neck, Indian Neck Heights, and Lieutenant Island. Sit here for a while and appreciate the merger of sea, sand, and sky, and a silence broken only by the cries of the birds. Now retrace your route to the parking area or, for an alternate return, walk back along the outer beach and then rejoin the described route via either of the two access trails at The Gut. (Please do not cut over the dunes or bushwhack through the forest, and remember that the access paths are closed at high tide during shorebird nesting season.)

ALTERNATE DIRECTIONS

From Route 6 southbound in Wellfleet, turn right at the first flashing yellow light and go 0.5 miles on Briar Lane to an intersection with West Main Street. Jog left on West Main Street; then immediately right on Holbrook Avenue. Continue straight on Holbrook Avenue 0.6 miles to Commercial Street. Bear right, go 0.1 mile to the Wellfleet Marina, and then follow the directions given on page 138.

Wellfleet and Truro Ponds

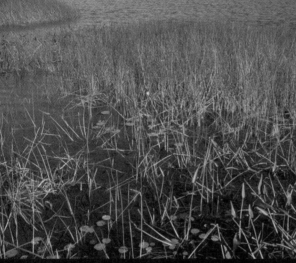

Ponds in Wellfleet and Truro, like most on Cape Cod, were formed by glacial activity.

KEY AT-A-GLANCE INFORMATION

GENERAL

DISTANCE 3.4 miles

TYPE OF WALK Loop

DIFFICULTY Moderate

TIME TO WALK 2–3 hours

MAPS *Cape Cod National Seashore,* National Geographic Maps; *Wellfleet,* USGS

SCENERY Forest, ponds

EXPOSURE TO SUN None

TRAIL TRAFFIC Light

TRAIL SURFACE(S) Dirt, sand

TRAILS OPEN All year

FEES/PASSES None

FACILITIES None

TRAIL USE

BICYCLES Allowed

DOGS Allowed on leash; not allowed in ponds or on pond beaches May 15–October 15

HUNTING Not allowed

HEALTH STATS

NUMBER OF STEPS 8,550

ESTIMATED CALORIES BURNED 407

DIRECTIONS TO TRAILHEAD

From Route 6 in Wellfleet, 1.1 mile north of a flashing yellow traffic signal and just opposite Pamet Point Road, go east on Black Pond Road, which is paved for a short distance and then becomes a single-lane, very rough dirt road with many driveways to private homes. Go 1.1 mile to a dirt road on the right, which leads about 50 feet to a dirt parking area. The trailhead is on the northeast corner of the parking area. (In summer, this parking area fills early with pond visitors.)

WALK SUMMARY

This athletic circuit passes seven kettle ponds that lie close to the Wellfleet–Truro line. Well shaded by towering pitch pines and a variety of other trees, enjoy this walk on a hot day or, even better, during the off-season, when the nearby vacation homes are empty and the pond shores silent. Although many of the dirt roads used to form this route have names, few are signed. This route passes many private homes; please respect private property and all postings.

DESCRIPTION

The parking area is perched on the Wellfleet–Truro line in a beautiful pine–oak forest. Due south is Wellfleet's Herring Pond, and just northeast is Truro's Slough Pond. Follow a 50-foot trail northeast to Black Pond Road and turn right. Be alert for cars.

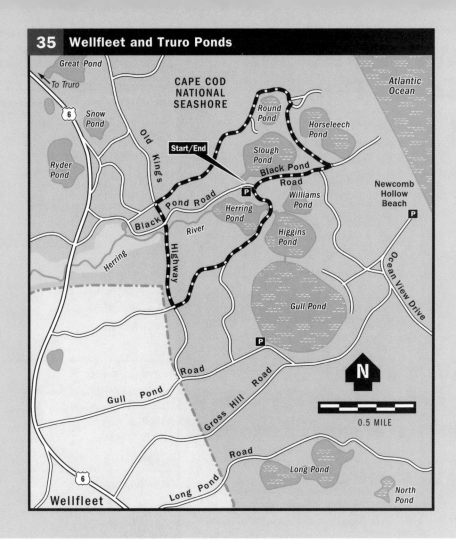

Great Pond

To Truro

CAPE COD
NATIONAL
SEASHORE

Atlantic
Ocean

6

Snow
Pond

Round
Pond

Horseleech
Pond

Old King's

Start/End

Slough
Pond

Black Pond

Ryder
Pond

Pond Road

Road

Newcomb
Hollow
Beach

Black

Herring
Pond

Williams
Pond

Higgins
Pond

Herring

River

Highway

Gull Pond

Road

N

Gull   Pond

Gross Hill   Road

0.5 MILE

Road

6

Long Pond

Long   Pond

Wellfleet

North
Pond

The road descends slightly, passes School House Hill Road, which is right, and then continues straight into Truro. There are a number of driveways and paths that diverge from the dirt roads used on this route: ignore them to remain on the described route.

After about 0.1 mile, a short, steep trail on your left provides access to Slough Pond. About 100 yards ahead, another trail, also right, leads past a rest bench to Slough Pond. Like most of the ponds on the Cape, the ponds on this route are in kettle holes—glacial depressions that intersect the water table. Their water levels rise and fall only through rainfall and evaporation, making them very susceptible to pollution.

Now the road climbs and offers glimpses through the trees of Williams Pond, to the right, one of four that connect to form the headwaters of Wellfleet's Herring River. During one of his trips to Cape Cod, Thoreau spent a night beside Williams Pond in a house belonging to John Newcomb, a self-described "poor good-for-thing crittur." The encounter furnished material for "The Wellfleet Oysterman" chapter in Thoreau's book *Cape Cod.* The road curves left, descends on a gentle grade, and then passes a driveway on the left signed CHERMAYEFF. After about 150 feet, a dirt road departs to the right. Walk another 250 feet or so and then veer sharply left on the next dirt road, Slough Pond Road (unsigned). There is a very small parking area here and a split-rail fence on the right.

Heading northwest, the road follows a rolling course with moderate grades—this is a hilly section of the Outer Cape. As you gain elevation, with driveways on the left and right, Horseleech Pond comes into view on the right. Cresting a rise, descend for about 100 yards to a fork, bear left for about 50 feet, and then merge with a dirt road joining from the right.

The road curves left around the north side of Round Pond, which is left, traversing a pine–oak forest with a dense, brushy understory. At about the 1-mile point, pass a trail departing to the right. Tracing the landscape's ups and downs, finally reach a high point, where a trail angles right. Stay on the road, curve left, and begin to descend. From a low point the road now makes a long, winding climb on a moderate grade. At the end of the climb, pass a trail cutting left into the understory and now enjoy a level stroll.

With power lines overhead, pass an overgrown dirt road joining from the right. Angle left and give up some of the hard-won elevation, passing dirt roads on the left and right. The gently curving descent soon levels, and you pass a house on the left. Go about 200 feet to a fork and veer left. Walk about 125 feet to the next junction; then angle left to merge with Old King's Highway, a dirt road. The "highway" is a historic track once used as a main route between Plymouth and Provincetown.

After about 150 feet meet a road departing left; continue straight to stay on Old King's Highway. Descend gently for another several hundred feet, cross Black Point Road (dirt), and continue straight. After about 75 feet, a short connector to Black Point Road joins from the left. Just ahead, at about the 2-mile point, the road dips to cross a culvert holding the mighty Herring River, which flows southeast, then south, before emptying into Wellfleet Harbor. Now on soft sand, climb moderately beneath tall pines, oaks, and black locusts, passing a driveway, which is left. At the next junction, where two closely spaced roads go right and soon join as one, stay straight on Old King's Highway.

Climb gently for another 200 feet or so; then descend to a four-way junction with a dirt road. Here turn left and, after several hundred feet, merge with a dirt road joining sharply from the right. Just ahead, pass a trail wandering right into the woods. Follow a sandy, gently rising course. Now angle slightly right and make a gentle descent, eventually merging with School House Hill Road, which joins from the right. Just ahead, pass a trail that angles left. Now descend for about150 feet to a fork. (From here, an 800-foot road, followed by a narrow, 200-foot trail, goes right, allowing you to explore the narrow barrier, cut by a sluice, between Gull and Higgins ponds. Pets are not allowed here.)

Bear left at the fork to stay on School House Hill Road, which curves left and is almost immediately joined on the right by a connector to the right branch of the previous fork. School House Hill Road runs along the barrier between Higgins and Herring ponds, but only Herring Pond is visible, to the left. There are short paths leading to each pond. Cresting a low rise, the road descends and then crosses a culvert, which carries water between the ponds. On a curvy, climbing course, soon turn left on a dirt road that enters the parking area from the east.

Bay View Trail and Fresh Brook Pathway

KEY AT-A-GLANCE INFORMATION

GENERAL

DISTANCE 1.9 miles

TYPE OF WALK Balloon

DIFFICULTY Moderate

TIME TO WALK 1–2 hours

MAPS Free handout from nature center; *Wellfleet*, USGS

SCENERY Forest, grassland, heathland, salt marsh

EXPOSURE TO SUN Partial

TRAIL TRAFFIC Light

TRAIL SURFACE(S) Dirt, sand, wood chips

TRAILS OPEN All year; 8 a.m.–sunset or until 8 p.m. in summer

FEES/PASSES Small fee for non-members of Massachusetts Audubon

FACILITIES Restrooms, water, nature center, butterfly garden, tent camping (members only)

TRAIL USE

BICYCLES Not allowed

DOGS Not allowed

HUNTING Not allowed

HEALTH STATS

NUMBER OF STEPS 4,275

ESTIMATED CALORIES BURNED 204

DIRECTIONS TO TRAILHEAD

From Route 6 in South Wellfleet, 1.5 miles south of the traffic signal at Marconi Beach Road, take West Road southwest 0.1 mile; then turn right on the sanctuary entrance road (single lane with turnouts). After 0.2 miles the road begins a one-way loop; parking and the nature center are just ahead. The trailhead is in front of the nature center. (Pay fee inside the nature center, or at a nearby self-registration station when the center is closed.)

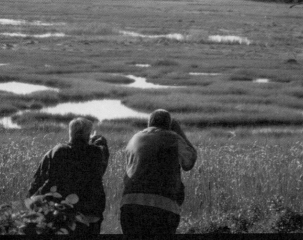

Birders near the start of the Bay View Trail use a spotting scope to scan the salt marsh.

WALK SUMMARY

Forest, marsh, heathland, and sandplain grassland communities all await you on this rewarding route, which also visits the glacial-outwash stream valley holding Fresh Brook. Although summer brings many people to this Massachusetts Audubon Society sanctuary, most opt for Goose Pond and the beach, so you can enjoy solitude by taking the trail less traveled. Opportunities for bird-watching and plant study abound. Visit the newly revamped nature center, which has displays and exhibits, a small gift shop and bookstore, and helpful, knowledgeable staff.

Note: Mass Audubon Wellfleet Bay Wildlife Sanctuary has an extensive program of classes, tours, guided walks, and summer programs for children; call (508) 349-2615 or visit **www.massaudubon .org/wellfleet** for more information.

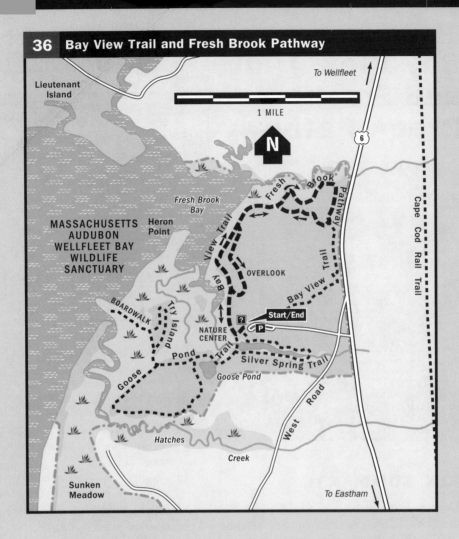

36 **Bay View Trail and Fresh Brook Pathway**

To Wellfleet

1 MILE

N

6

Lieutenant
Island

Fresh Brook
Bay

Fresh Brook Pathway

MASSACHUSETTS
AUDUBON
WELLFLEET BAY
WILDLIFE
SANCTUARY

Heron
Point

Bay View Trail

OVERLOOK

Bay View Trail

Cape Cod Rail Trail

BOARDWALK

Try Island

Start/End

P

NATURE
CENTER

Pond
Trail

Goose Pond

Silver Spring Trail

Goose Pond

West Road

Hatches

Creek

Sunken
Meadow

To Eastham

DESCRIPTION

Following the Goose Pond Trail, surfaced from here to Goose Pond to accommodate wheelchairs and strollers, walk south beside the nature center about
100 feet to a junction. Here the Silver Spring Trail goes straight, but turn right,
passing an information board, and go about hundred feet to a junction. Now
bear right on the Bay View Trail. Ahead is a large expanse of salt marsh, with
some areas freshened by Silver Spring Brook, which flows into the marsh a few
hundred yards south of here. Try Island, named for the large pots used to render whale blubber, is across the marsh to the west.

FLORA

The sanctuary is a plant-lover's paradise. Some of the common trees on this route include pitch pine, black oak, white oak, black cherry, eastern red cedar, black locust, and shadbush. The marsh hosts saltwater cordgrass, salt hay, sea lavender, glasswort, common and narrow-leaved cattails, and common reed. Along the upper edge of the marsh, look for groundsel tree and marsh elder. Shrubs such as bearberry, black huckleberry, poverty grass, golden heather, bayberry, scrub oak, beach plum, and smooth sumac favor dry, sandy areas. In season, wildflowers decorate the hillsides.

FAUNA

In wooded areas, look for woodpeckers, black-capped chickadees, tufted titmice, nuthatches, and warblers. Herons and egrets inhabit the marshes. Shorebirds feeding in the marsh may include whimbrels, black-bellied plovers, short-billed dowitchers, yellowlegs, and various sandpipers. Cooper's hawks and peregrine falcons may be patrolling the skies.

The trail curves right and runs between a wooded upland, right, and the cattail-fringed marsh, left. Passing a rest bench, right, enjoy a level walk and soon reach a clearing, where you can view the marsh up close. Now angling away from the marsh, climb gently through an avenue of black locusts (trees, not bugs!) to a T-junction. Turn left, stroll through a shrubby corridor, pass a couple of rest benches, and descend to the marsh.

A sandy, level trail skirts the marsh through a zone flooded by only the highest tides. After about 0.5 miles, turn right and go about 30 feet to a T-junction. Turn left, pass a rest bench, and arrive at a junction with the Fresh Brook Pathway loop. Bear left and climb into a forest bordering Fresh Brook, which gets its start in Cape Cod National Seashore near the Atlantic Ocean, flows under Route 6, and empties into Wellfleet Harbor near Lieutenant Island, thus nearly bisecting the Cape at one of its narrower points. Several rest benches provide viewing opportunities.

The trail follows a curvy, rolling course beside Fresh Brook, then turns right and climbs moderately through forest to a T-junction. Here, turn right, descend gently beside pines and oaks, and then close the loop at the junction with the Bay View Trail. Now retrace your route on the Bay View Trail to the next junction, where you go straight, following a sign for the nature center. With the marsh to your right, curve left and climb moderately to a heathland, where the best views so far await, along with a rest bench.

Now descend and curve right, passing a sandplain grassland, left, studded with blue-bird boxes on poles. At a T-junction, where a closed trail to the day-camp area goes left, you turn right. After about 150 feet reach a junction signed for the nature center. Turn left and retrace your route to the parking area.

KEY AT-A-GLANCE INFORMATION

GENERAL

DISTANCE 1.4 miles

TYPE OF WALK Balloon

DIFFICULTY Easy

TIME TO WALK 1–2 hours

MAPS Free handout from nature center; *Wellfleet,* USGS

SCENERY Forest, pond, salt marsh

EXPOSURE TO SUN Partial

TRAIL TRAFFIC Heavy

TRAIL SURFACE(S) Dirt, sand, wood chips

TRAILS OPEN All year; 8 a.m.–sunset or until 8 p.m. in summer

FEES/PASSES Small fee for non-members of Massachusetts Audubon

FACILITIES Restrooms, water, nature center, butterfly garden, tent camping

TRAIL USE

BICYCLES Not allowed

DOGS Not allowed

HUNTING Not allowed

HEALTH STATS

NUMBER OF STEPS 3,150

ESTIMATED CALORIES BURNED 150

DIRECTIONS TO TRAILHEAD

From Route 6 in South Wellfleet, 1.5 miles south of the traffic signal at Marconi Beach Road, take West Road southwest 0.1 mile; then turn right on the sanctuary entrance road (single lane with turnouts). After 0.2 miles the road begins a one-way loop; parking and the nature center are just ahead. The trailhead is in front of the nature center. (Pay fee inside the nature center, or at a nearby self-registration station when the center is closed.)

Goose Pond Trail

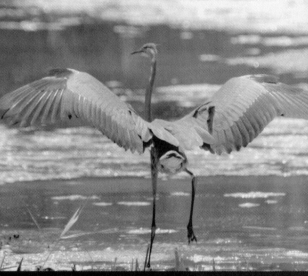

Goose Pond is a great place to watch birds, such as this great blue heron.

WALK SUMMARY

The first part of the self-guided Goose Pond Trail, from the nature center to Goose Pond, is an "all person accessible" trail, designed to accommodate wheelchairs and strollers. Beyond Goose Pond the route follows a well-trodden path out to a salt marsh. At the marsh most folks leave the self-guided trail and walk via a path and boardwalks to a beach on Wellfleet Harbor. Your route stays on the Goose Pond Trail as it skirts the marsh and then loops back through open and then wooded country to Goose Pond and back to the nature center. The variety of native plants and the chance to see and hear many of the Cape's common (and not-so-common) birds make this walk a must-do. Parts of the route may flood during very high tides.

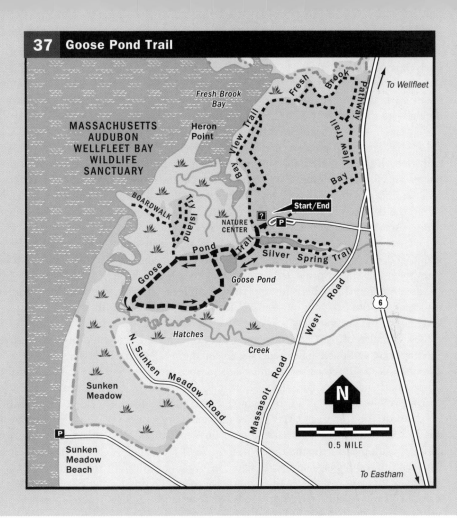

Be sure to visit the newly revamped, state-of-the-environmental-art nature center, which has displays and exhibits, a small gift shop/bookstore, and helpful, knowledgeable staff. There you can buy or borrow a trail guide; numbered markers along the trail, indicated by boldface numbers in the description below, are keyed to text in the guide.

Note: Mass Audubon Wellfleet Bay Wildlife Sanctuary has an extensive program of classes, tours, guided walks, and summer programs for children; call (508) 349-2615 or visit **www.massaudubon.org/wellfleet** for details.

DESCRIPTION

To begin, follow the self-guided Goose Pond Trail, surfaced from here to the Goose Pond to accommodate wheelchairs and strollers, south between the nature center and the butterfly garden about 100 feet to a junction. Here the Silver Spring Trail goes straight, but turn right, passing an information board and then marker **1,** for pitch pine. Go about 50 feet to a junction and marker **2,** for panic grass. Where the Bay View Trail veers right, you continue straight, passing marker **3,** which indicates nonnative plants such as trumpet vine and Japanese honeysuckle. Now pass a short connector, on the right, to the Bay View Trail.

Marker **4** is for people and the landscape. A dam across Silver Spring Brook, just ahead, has created a pond, which is now a haven for wildlife. Soon you meet a short path, left, leading to a boardwalk overlooking the pond, where markers **5,** wetland plants, and **6,** turtles, await. Eastern painted turtles are frequently seen from the boardwalk, sunning themselves on a log, as are dragonflies, damselflies, and songbirds. Just before the dam's spillway, pass marker **7,** for Silver Spring Brook. Look nearby for evidence—scat and worn areas, or slides—of river otters.

Now cross the dam—a salt marsh is to your right—and find marker **8,** for red maple and white poplar; marker **9,** for amphibians; and marker **10,** for winterberry. Soon meet the Silver Spring Trail, which departs left. Black-capped chickadees, marker **11,** are common throughout the sanctuary. Continue straight on a sandy path carpeted with pine needles, passing marker **12,** for lichens; marker **13,** for common hairgrass; and marker **14,** for poison ivy.

Like much of the Cape, this area was once denuded, but it has been reforested to check erosion and provide food and shelter for animals. Marker **15** highlights three of the four pine species found on the sanctuary. At an open area bordered by a split-rail fence, the Goose Pond Trail turns right and a short trail to an observation/photography blind goes straight. Follow the trail as it turns right and reaches a boardwalk beside Goose Pond.

Goose Pond, marker **16,** is one of the sanctuary's prime bird-watching spots. The pond's level is adjusted seasonally to meet the needs of different animals. During spring and early summer, for example, the water is kept fairly high to benefit Fowler's toads. Later, as the southward shorebird migration begins in mid-July, the water level is lowered to expose some of the pond's muddy shoreline. During the daily cycle of tides, the water in nearby Wellfleet Harbor floods sandbars and mudflats where shorebirds feed and roost. Some of these birds find sanctuary in Goose Pond and in the adjacent salt marsh, particularly at or near high tide.

Cross the boardwalk, where there are several rest benches and a "window" through the vegetation to the pond. Marker **17** is for the cattails and phragmites, or common reeds, that fringe the pond. Marker **18** indicates two very different mammals, bats and muskrats, which may be seen here. Marker **19,** just past the pond, is for groundsel tree, a plant of the salt marsh's upper edge.

Now back in forest, meet marker **20,** for black racer, a type of snake. Here a path on your right leads to another active bird-watching spot and marker **21.** Beyond marker **21** is an opening in the salt marsh called a salt panne, caused by the lethal effect on marsh grasses of evaporated salt from extremely high tides. The resulting shallow, grass-free pool attracts shorebirds at high tide.

Continuing westward on the Goose Pond Trail, pass marker **22,** for two species of greenbrier. At a junction just ahead, the return part of the self-guided trail joins on the left. Also here are marker **23,** for asparagus, once a local crop; and marker **24,** for

FLORA

All the usual arboreal suspects—pitch pine, black oak, white oak, black cherry, and eastern red cedar—are here, along with conifers brought in for reforestation during the 1930s, when the area was being used as an ornithological research station. Hickory, black locust, sassafras, bayberry, beach plum, scrub oak, dwarf chestnut oak, and smooth sumac also dot the dry, sandy soil.

Salt-marsh plants here include saltwater cordgrass, salt hay, glasswort, sea lavender, sea blite, marsh elder, and groundsel tree. Common and narrow-leaved cattails, along with common reed, an invasive nonnative species, border fresh and brackish water. Ground cover and vines include bearberry, broom crowberry, poison ivy, Virginia creeper, wild grape, bullbrier, and catbrier. Wildflowers are plentiful in season.

FAUNA

Some of the mammals seen here include rabbits, chipmunks, gray squirrels, and coyotes. Reptiles and amphibians include snakes, turtles, frogs, and toads. Frisky fiddler crabs entertain young and old alike.

The real stars, however, are the many different species of birds that nest here or pass through on migration. Among these are songbirds such as the black-capped chickadee, American goldfinch, eastern towhee, northern mockingbird, blue jay, red-winged blackbird, belted kingfisher, tree swallow, northern bobwhite, and various woodpeckers, warblers, and sparrows.

Wading birds include green heron, great blue heron, great egret, and snowy egret. The sanctuary's impressive list of shorebirds includes black-bellied plover, semipalmated plover, piping plover, American oystercatcher, whimbrel, greater yellowlegs, lesser yellowlegs, pectoral sandpiper, stilt sandpiper, solitary sandpiper, spotted sandpiper, semipalmated sandpiper, and least sandpiper, not to mention rarities from abroad. Cooper's hawks and peregrine falcons are several of the raptors seen here.

butterfly weed and butterflies. Eastern red cedar, marker **25,** is one of the first trees to spread into formerly open fields.

Now pass an observation deck, marker **26,** that offers fine views of Wellfleet Harbor, which is bounded on the west by Great Island and Jeremy Point, both part of Cape Cod National Seashore. The low rise just across the marsh is called Try Island, named for the large pots used to render whale blubber. The trail now passes a hillside, left, where sanctuary staff have used fire and other management techniques to restore a heathland habitat. Marker **27** highlights bearberry, a heathland plant. Marker **28** is for crickets and grasshoppers. Two of the sanctuary's common birds, northern mockingbird and prairie warbler, may be seen and heard near marker **29.**

Nearing a large salt marsh, pass markers **30,** for wild grapes, and **31,** for sassafras. Now stroll to a T-junction on the edge of the salt marsh, indicated by marker **32.** Here a trail to Try Island and the beach goes right, but turn left instead to stay on the Goose Pond Trail. Follow a wide, sandy path southwest beside the marsh. The highest tides, around the full and new moons, flood this part of the route. Marker **33** indicates fiddler crabs, whose antics as they scurry to and fro delight children and adults alike. Marker **34** is for some of the salt-marsh plants, which you can study here up close. Birds of the salt marsh, marker **35,** include shorebirds and raptors. Tides, marker **36,** are the lifeblood of the marsh.

At about the 0.5-mile point, a sign directs you left, away from the marsh, on a sandy trail. The change in vegetation is sudden and striking: instead of low-growing, salt-tolerant plants, there are upland trees and shrubs, including beach plum, marker **37**. Climbing slightly, merge with a dirt road that joins sharply from the left, and pass marker **38**, for diamondback terrapin, a salt-marsh turtle that is state-listed as a threatened species. Marker **39**, nearby, is for little bluestem grass. Now stroll by marker **40**, for goldenrods and asters, whose numerous species provide late summer and fall color.

Several inviting rest benches, right, overlook a salt marsh bordering Hatches Creek. Beyond them is marker **41**, for American kestrel, the smallest North American falcon. The open fields to the left of the road are more examples of restored heathland habitat.

Leave the dirt road where directed by a sign for the nature center. Follow a sandy single-track trail into forest, passing marker **42**, for sickle-leaved golden aster. Nearby are marker **43**, for northern bayberry; marker **44**, for a hillside carpeted with broom crow-berry, state-listed as a species of special concern; and marker **45**, for Cape Cod woodlands. The final cluster of markers—**46**, **47**, **48**, and **49**—are for scrub oak, black oak, black huckleberry, and two species of heather (Hudsonia), or poverty grass.

After passing Goose Pond, right, which is mostly hidden by a screen of trees and shrubs, close the loop at a T-junction. Now turn right and retrace your route to the parking area.

Bearberry Hill and Bog House

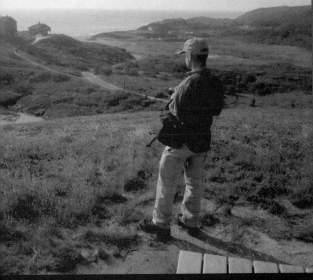

Bearberry Hill provides a sweeping view of Truro's Atlantic coastline.

WALK SUMMARY

Views of the Atlantic Ocean from Bearberry Hill, along with a visit to a cranberry bog and the restored Bog House, highlight this short loop through the Truro hills. Asters and goldenrods blooming in late summer and fall add a dash of color to the route.

DESCRIPTION

From the parking area, follow a dirt trail north a few hundred feet to North Pamet Road (ignore the unofficial trail heading southwest). Carefully cross the road, climb a few concrete steps, and turn left on a dirt trail signed for the Pamet Valley and Bearberry Hill trails. At a junction with a closed trail, turn right on the dirt-and-gravel Bearberry Hill Trail. Emerging from forest, traverse a

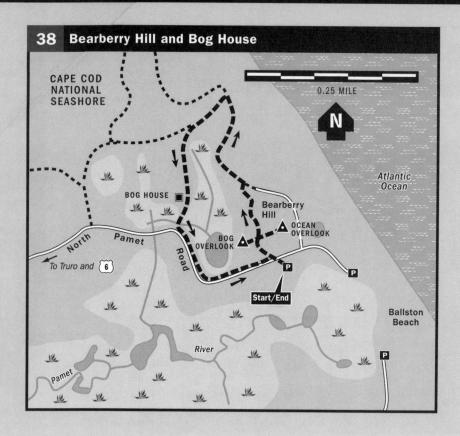

bearberry-covered hillside, gaining views of the Atlantic Ocean and the marshy headwaters of the Pamet River.

At a fork, bear right on a sandy trail to visit the Ocean Overlook, which sits atop a large hill. Blasts of wind from the ocean ensure that only the hardiest plants—stunted forms of pitch pine, eastern red cedar, black cherry, and bayberry—cling to the hillside. From the overlook, a wooden platform, you have superb 360-degree views.

Now retrace your route to the previous junction and turn right. Go about 100 feet to the next junction: from here, the Bog Overlook is straight and the Bog House Trail is right. Walk straight on a sandy trail to a wooden platform, which affords a fine view of the Bog House, a cranberry bog, and a large pond fringed with shrubs. After enjoying the view, return to the previous junction and turn left on the gravel Bog House Trail.

Wind downhill on a moderate grade, aided in places by steps. After the trail levels, curve right and climb to a T-junction with a sandy path, signed bog house, left, parking lot, right. Turn left and soon reach a junction with the Bog House Trail. Turn left on a sandy single-track trail and cross on open area dotted

FLORA	FAUNA
Bearberry, also called hog cranberry because of its unpalatable red berries, is a member of the heath family. Other heath-family members found here include black huckleberry, highbush blueberry, and cranberry. Pitch pine, black oak, scrub oak, black cherry, beach plum, and bayberry grow beside the trail, as do asters and goldenrods.	American goldfinches, tree swallows, gray catbirds, northern flickers, eastern kingbirds, and blue jays are some of birds you may see and hear from the trail.

with wind-pruned trees. However, as you travel farther from the ocean, the effects of the wind lessen, and the tree cover thickens.

Where an unsigned trail goes straight, angle left and follow a rolling course through an area dense with trees and shrubs. A step-aided descent soon brings you to the Bog House, where a restoration project by the Friends of Cape Cod National Seashore has spruced up the 1830s building and will restore the adjacent cranberry bog. A nearby information panel, beside the bog, describes the ecology of the wild cranberry and its traditional use by Native Americans and the Pilgrims.

From here, walk between the house (right) and the bog (left) to find a grassy dirt road. Follow it to North Pamet Road; then turn left and walk along the road's left side (facing traffic) for about 0.4 miles to close the loop at the concrete steps. Carefully cross North Pamet Road and retrace your route to the parking area.

GENERAL

DISTANCE 3.7 miles

TYPE OF WALK Loop

DIFFICULTY Moderate

TIME TO WALK 2–3 hours

MAPS *North Truro,* USGS

SCENERY Atlantic Ocean, hills, forest

EXPOSURE TO SUN Partial

TRAIL TRAFFIC Light

TRAIL SURFACE(S) Dirt, gravel, sand, pavement

TRAILS OPEN All year

FEES/PASSES None

FACILITIES None

TRAIL USE

BICYCLES Allowed

DOGS Allowed on leash

HUNTING Not allowed

HEALTH STATS

NUMBER OF STEPS 8,325

ESTIMATED CALORIES BURNED 396

DIRECTIONS TO TRAILHEAD

From Route 6 northbound in Truro, take the Pamet Roads–Truro Center exit. After 100 feet, turn left on North Pamet Road. Go 1.5 miles; then turn right on a driveway (just past a roadside parking area and just before a youth hostel). Now turn immediately right into a small parking area. From 9 a.m. to 6 p.m., parking here is limited to 2 hours. The trailhead is on the northwest side of the parking area, beside a CCNS information board.

From Route 6 southbound in Truro, take the Pamet Roads–Truro Center exit. After exiting, bear right and go 0.1 mile to an intersection signed for Pamet Roads, Route 6, and Provincetown. Turn right, go under Route 6, and at the next intersection turn left on North Pamet Road. After several hundred feet, the exit from Route 6 northbound joins at left. From here, follow directions above.

Truro Hills

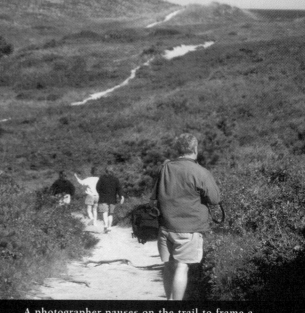

A photographer pauses on the trail to frame a picture of the Truro Hills.

WALK SUMMARY

This scenic, mostly shady circuit in the Truro Hills has something for everyone—vistas of the Atlantic Ocean to admire, a wide variety of native plants to study, birds to see and hear. Part of the route follows a segment of Old King's Highway, a historic track that was once the main route between Plymouth and Provincetown.

DESCRIPTION

From the parking area, follow a dirt trail north a few hundred feet to North Pamet Road (ignore the unofficial trail heading southwest). Turn right on the road, staying along its left side (facing traffic). After about 100 yards, you turn left on a dirt-and-gravel road that climbs on a moderate grade across the base of Bearberry Hill, over to your left. The

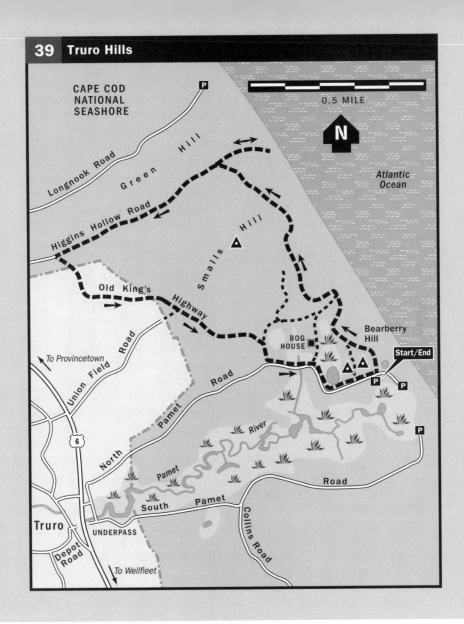

CAPE COD
NATIONAL
SEASHORE

Longnook Road

Green Hill

Higgins Hollow Road

Old King's Highway

Smalls Hill

0.5 MILE

N

Atlantic
Ocean

To Provincetown

Union Field Road

To Wellfleet

Truro

UNDERPASS

Depot Road

North Pamet Road

Pamet

South Pamet

Collins Road

Pamet River

BOG HOUSE

Bearberry Hill

Start/End

Road

Atlantic Ocean to your right is hidden by sea cliffs, but later you will enjoy views of it from a fine vantage point.

The road levels, curves left, and then descends through a forest of pitch pines. Where the road bends sharply right, walk straight on a dirt fire road, passing left of a cable that blocks vehicle access. About 100 yards ahead, the Bearberry Hill Trail joins from the left. In late summer and fall, this is one of the most colorful spots on the Outer Cape, with purple asters and yellow goldenrods set

159

FLORA	FAUNA
Plant enthusiasts have plenty to study here. Trees include pitch pine, black cherry, black oak, white oak, white poplar, bigtooth aspen, black locust, and shadbush. Some of the shrubs growing beside the route are bearberry, black huckleberry, lowbush blueberry, broom crowberry, bayberry, beach plum, arrowwood, scrub oak, dwarf chestnut oak, dwarf sumac, and winterberry. Goldenrods, asters, Virginia creeper, and poison ivy add color in late summer and fall.	Be alert for forest birds, including blue jays, catbirds, and northern flickers. In more open areas, look for American goldfinches, tree swallows, and eastern kingbirds.

against a dark-green background of bearberry, with burgundy leaves of Virginia creeper added for good measure.

Soon the Bog House Trail departs left, but go straight another 50 feet or so to a fork. Stay left, and follow a sandy trail that curves left and climbs moderately. This is true wilderness, protected from development as part of the Cape Cod National Seashore. Along the way, several unsigned trails depart from the main route: ignore them to stay on the described route. Now the grade eases, and you enjoy a mostly level walk on a dirt trail, for a while squeezing through a narrow corridor of scrub oak. Another moderate climb and then a level stretch bring you to a T-junction with a paved road.

Turn right and climb to a terrific vantage point, where two rest benches and views of the Atlantic Ocean, fronted by towering sea cliffs, await. Like many of the Cape's other landforms, the cliffs owe their existence to glacial activity, combined with erosion from waves and wind. After enjoying this special spot, return to the previous junction and continue straight (the pavement ends after several hundred yards). Descend moderately, now on dirt and sand, and soon reach level ground. As you retreat from the ocean's edge to more sheltered ground, the pines and oaks become taller.

After passing a dirt road on the left and an unsigned trail to Long Nook Road on the right, reach paved Higgins Hollow Road. Walk straight—past a dirt road, left, and a driveway, right—then turn left on a dirt road signed with the names of homeowners. This is part of Old King's Highway, thought to have begun as a Native American route. In colonial days, it became the Cape's main thoroughfare from Plymouth to Provincetown. (The road passes private homes; please respect private property.)

Climbing on a gentle grade, pass straight through several junctions, including one with a road, on your right, signed 4TH OF JULY RD., PRIVATE WAY. Enjoy a shady walk, in some places on soft sand, soon passing a gravel driveway signed SECREST 54, angling right. Climb past a house with a lovely garden, crest a rise, and begin to descend. Go straight through a four-way junction, where a dirt road goes right and a trail departs left. Several hundred feet ahead, pass an overgrown dirt road on your right.

Climbing again, meet more roads departing left and right, but continue straight. When you reach paved North Pamet Road, turn left and walk along its left side (facing traffic). Soon pass the road to the Bog House, left, and walk another 0.4 miles to close the loop at the concrete steps. Carefully cross North Pamet Road and retrace your route to the parking area.

Pilgrim Spring Trail

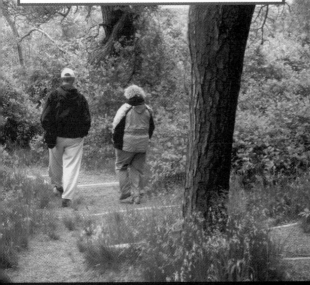

Pilgrim Spring Trail visits the spot where the Pilgrims first found fresh water.

KEY AT-A-GLANCE INFORMATION

GENERAL

DISTANCE 0.7 miles

TYPE OF WALK Loop

DIFFICULTY Easy

TIME TO WALK 1 hour or less

MAPS *Cape Cod National Seashore,* National Geographic Maps; *North Truro,* USGS

SCENERY Dunes, forest, marsh

EXPOSURE TO SUN Partial

TRAIL TRAFFIC Moderate

TRAIL SURFACE(S) Dirt, pavement

TRAILS OPEN All year

FEES/PASSES None

FACILITIES Restrooms and water (seasonal); picnic tables, interpretive shelter

TRAIL USE

BICYCLES Not allowed

DOGS Not allowed

HUNTING Not allowed

HEALTH STATS

NUMBER OF STEPS 1,575

ESTIMATED CALORIES BURNED 75

DIRECTIONS TO TRAILHEAD

From the intersection of Routes 6 and 6A in North Truro, take Route 6 north for 2.1 miles; then turn right on an unnamed road signed PILGRIM HEIGHTS. Go 0.4 miles to a large, paved parking area on the left side of a one-way loop. Two trails depart from a trailhead at the northwest side of the one-way loop. The trail to Small's Swamp goes northwest, toward the interpretive shelter. A short trail to Pilgrim Spring veers right (northeast) from the trail to the shelter. (The restrooms, water, and picnic tables are a short distance south, adjacent to the next parking area.)

WALK SUMMARY

Where the Pilgrims first found fresh water, you can enjoy a quiet ramble amid a variety of native trees and shrubs on this short, easy loop. Trailside markers identify some of the common plants. (While here, also visit the Small's Swamp Trail, which departs from the same trailhead as the trail to Pilgrim Spring.)

DESCRIPTION

Just before reaching the interpretive shelter, veer right on a dirt trail and enjoy a level, forested walk. On a curvy course, descend gently to an overlook, where the view extends eastward across a freshwater marsh to a line of dunes. A narrow corridor of shrubs leads to a clearing with a picnic table.

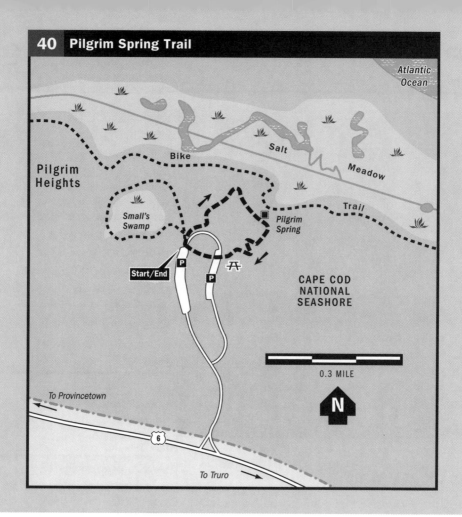

Nearby, less than a week after making landfall in Provincetown, a party of Pilgrims found their first supply of fresh water.

With a bike trail on your left, turn right and climb a trail carpeted with pine needles. The pines here are venerable elders, their limbs twisted with age and exposure to the elements. After a switchback and a moderate ascent, find level ground amid the pines. Soon reach a paved path that skirts some restrooms and leads through a picnic area. When you reach a large parking area, cross it and find the continuation of the trail, now a level dirt track. When you reach a grassy area, climb an embankment to reach the east side of the first parking area.

FLORA

Pitch pine, scrub oak, black cherry, arrowwood, bayberry, beach plum, highbush blueberry, lowbush blueberry, salt-spray rose, and winterberry add botanical interest to the route. The ever-present poison ivy is here, as are bullbrier, Virginia creeper, blackberry, honeysuckle, and wild sarsaparilla.

KEY AT-A-GLANCE INFORMATION

GENERAL

DISTANCE 0.8 miles

TYPE OF WALK Balloon

DIFFICULTY Easy

TIME TO WALK 1 hour or less

MAPS *Cape Cod National Seashore,* National Geographic Maps; *North Truro,* USGS

SCENERY Atlantic Ocean, kettle hole, dunes

EXPOSURE TO SUN Partial

TRAIL TRAFFIC Moderate

TRAIL SURFACE(S) Dirt, pavement

TRAILS OPEN All year

FEES/PASSES None

FACILITIES Restrooms and water (seasonal); picnic tables, interpretive shelter

TRAIL USE

BICYCLES Not allowed

DOGS Not allowed

HUNTING Not allowed

HEALTH STATS

NUMBER OF STEPS 1,800

ESTIMATED CALORIES BURNED 86

DIRECTIONS TO TRAILHEAD

From the intersection of Routes 6 and 6A in North Truro, take Route 6 north for 2.1 miles; then turn right on an unnamed road signed PILGRIM HEIGHTS. Go 0.4 miles to a large, paved parking area on the left side of a one-way loop. Two trails depart from a trailhead at the northwest side of the one-way loop. The trail to Small's Swamp goes northwest, toward the interpretive shelter. A trail to Pilgrim Spring veers right (northeast) from the trail to the shelter. (The restrooms, water, and picnic tables are a short distance south, adjacent to the next parking area.)

Small's Swamp Trail

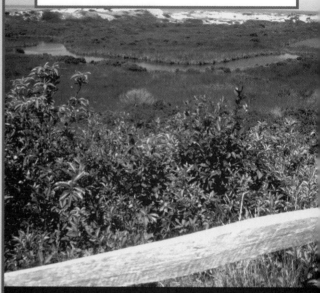

View north from Small's Swamp Trail reveals freshwater marsh, dunes, and the Atlantic Ocean.

WALK SUMMARY

Short in length but rich in history and plant life, this loop around Small's Swamp, at the bottom of a glacial kettle hole, is a rewarding walk back in time. Native Americans, the newcomers aboard the *Mayflower,* and 19th-century farmers all had a stake in this little plot of ground, which is now preserved for us to enjoy. Trailside markers identify some of the common plants. (While here, also visit the Pilgrim Spring Trail, which departs from the same trailhead as the trail to Small's Swamp.)

DESCRIPTION

Before starting your walk, visit the shelter beside the trailhead and view interpretive panels describing the three discovery trips made by parties from the *Mayflower,* which anchored on November 11, 1620,

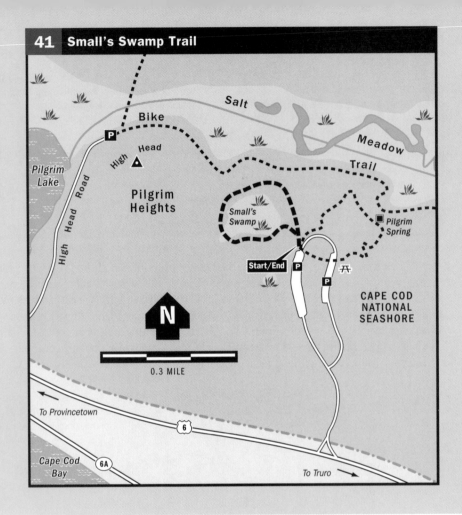

in nearby Provincetown. The kettle hole in view to the northwest was used by Native Americans, and artifacts found there are more than 7,000 years old. In the 1860s, Thomas Small established a 200-acre farm amid an otherwise barren landscape.

Via a log-bordered trail, descend on a moderate grade into a shady, cool pine forest. After about 100 yards the trail forks. Stay left, following a split-rail fence. The route swings sharply left and brings you to the swamp, which occupies the floor of the kettle hole that is visible from the shelter. A short boardwalk takes you across the possibly wet area. Now climbing on a gentle grade, the trail traverses a shrubby zone and soon brings you to a vantage point, where views of the Atlantic Ocean and a freshwater marsh await. The ecology of the surrounding area changed after 1869, when a dike—which is now the roadbed for Route 6—enclosed Provincetown's East Harbor and created Pilgrim Lake, cutting off tidal flow from Cape Cod Bay.

FLORA	FAUNA
Although short, this walk visits several different habitats with an impressive variety of plants. The forest is typical of the Outer Cape, with pitch pine, black oak, scrub oak, black cherry, and bayberry. In Small's Swamp, look for highbush blueberry, swamp azalea, sweet pepperbush, arrowwood, and winterberry. Ground cover includes bearberry, poison ivy, Virginia creeper, lowbush blueberry, and wild sarsaparilla. There are even some trees, such as domestic apple, left over from the area's farming days.	Red-winged blackbirds, blue jays, and sparrows are all at home here. Don't be surprised to spot coyote scat or tracks; these predators are now common on the Cape.

If you hear voices in the distance, they're not from Pilgrim ghosts. A popular bicycle trail, which runs between High Head and Head of the Meadow, is between here and the dunes to the east. About 100 yards from the first vantage point is another overlook—an interpretive panel, once here but now gone told the story of the British man-of-war *Somerset*, which in 1778 went aground on Peaked Hills Bar, a shallow shoal just offshore that has trapped many ships. Now returning to forest, soon close the loop, bear left, and retrace your route to the parking area.

Beech Forest Trail

KEY AT-A-GLANCE INFORMATION

GENERAL

DISTANCE 1.2 miles

TYPE OF WALK Loop

DIFFICULTY Easy

TIME TO WALK 1 hour or less

MAPS *Beech Forest Trail*, CCNS brochure with map; *Cape Cod National Seashore*, National Geographic Maps; *Provincetown*, USGS

SCENERY Dunes, forest, ponds, wetlands

EXPOSURE TO SUN Partial

TRAIL TRAFFIC Moderate

TRAIL SURFACE(S) Dirt, sand

TRAILS OPEN All year

FEES/PASSES None

FACILITIES Restrooms, water, picnic tables

TRAIL USE

BICYCLES Not allowed

DOGS Not allowed

HUNTING Not allowed

HEALTH STATS

NUMBER OF STEPS 3,150

ESTIMATED CALORIES BURNED 150

DIRECTIONS TO TRAILHEAD

From Route 6 in Provincetown, take Race Point Road northwest 0.5 miles; then turn left on the Beech Forest entrance road. Go several hundred feet to a fork and bear right. There are 2 parking areas: one just past the fork, the other just past where the entrance road loops left. The trailhead is on the northeast side of the first parking area.

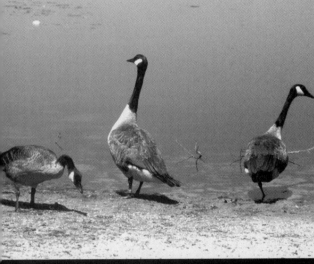

Canada geese often gather beside the parking area near the start of the Beech Forest Trail.

WALK SUMMARY

This classic stroll, which loops around a freshwater wetland and visits a secluded American beech forest, is perfect for nature lovers. Plant enthusiasts will enjoy the variety of trees and shrubs, many of them identified by trailside markers. Birders visiting in spring and fall should be on the lookout for migrating warblers and other songbirds. There is a brochure with a map available at the trailhead. Mosquitoes are plentiful here in summer.

DESCRIPTION

To begin, take an elevated boardwalk through a shady, swampy area that is part of a large freshwater wetland made up of several ponds and marshes. Cattails fringe the ponds, which host a variety of vegetation, including pickerelweed and white water

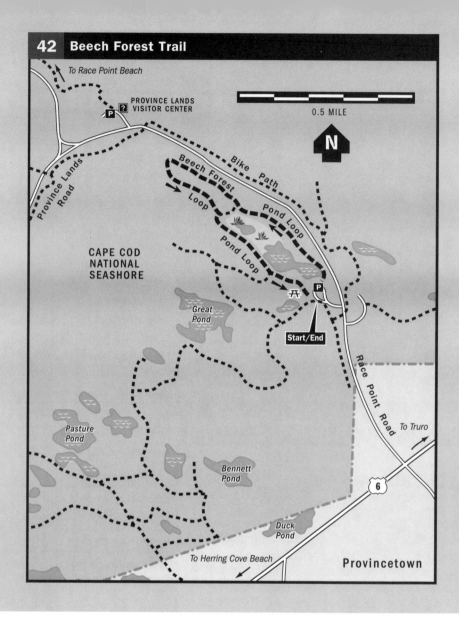

To Race Point Beach

PROVINCE LANDS
VISITOR CENTER

0.5 MILE

N

Bike Path

Beech Forest
Loop

Pond Loop

Pond Loop

Province Lands Road

CAPE COD
NATIONAL
SEASHORE

Great
Pond

Start/End

Race Point Road

To Truro

Pasture
Pond

Bennett
Pond

6

Duck
Pond

To Herring Cove Beach

Provincetown

lilies. Hidden among the vegetation, a chorus of frogs may greet you. For most of the year, this walk sees a moderate number of visitors. But during the warbler migration, especially early on a May morning, be prepared to meet lots of avid birders, bubbling with enthusiasm over the latest sightings. This forest is one of the few wooded areas on the Cape's otherwise exposed tip and serves as a haven for birds.

After about 100 yards, leave the boardwalk and access a sandy trail that skirts a vast system of sand dunes. The trail, level at first, now climbs. The wetland to your left is screened from view by trees and shrubs. In places, the sand is soft and the trail is exposed to the sun. Soon, however, regain shade and find the first American beech trees, identified by their large papery, serrated leaves with prominent veins, and smooth light-gray bark.

At about 0.5 miles, reach a junction. (To shorten the walk, turn left here and follow the route description from the next junction, below.) Continue straight, now in a deep ravine filled with American beech. The light filtering through the beech leaves enhances the magical quality of the cool, refreshing forest. Before European settlement, forests of beech and other hardwoods were common on the Cape. By the mid-1800s, when Thoreau visited, many of the trees had been cut, leaving large swaths of land subject to erosion. Reforestation and natural forest succession have returned the Cape to a mostly wooded state.

When you reach a fence, turn sharply left and climb a steep set of dirt steps braced by logs, leaving behind the beech trees. Briefly atop a ridge, turn right and descend, aided again by dirt steps. After a rolling course brings you to a fork, bear right and enjoy a fine view of the wetland to your left. Dunes rise steeply to your right—this forest, here mostly pitch pine, is an island in a sea of sand.

Two unsigned paths, not part of the trail system, join from the right, but you continue straight. A third path, also right, leads a few hundred feet to a boardwalk that extends over a pond. From there, you can examine the pond and wetland plants up close, study dragonflies, and croak to the frogs. Back on the main trail, cross a swampy area on a boardwalk, and then reach a paved path, which immediately forks. Restrooms and water are to your right; the parking areas are several hundred feet to your left.

GENERAL

DISTANCE 6.6 miles

TYPE OF WALK Balloon

DIFFICULTY Difficult

TIME TO WALK 3–5 hours

MAPS *Cape Cod National Seashore,* National Geographic Maps; *Provincetown,* USGS

SCENERY Provincetown Harbor and waterfront, lighthouses, Cape Cod Bay

EXPOSURE TO SUN Full

TRAIL TRAFFIC Moderate

TRAIL SURFACE(S) Rock, sand

TRAILS OPEN All year

FEES/PASSES None

FACILITIES None

TRAIL USE

BICYCLES Not allowed

DOGS Allowed on leash

HUNTING Not allowed

HEALTH STATS

NUMBER OF STEPS 14,850

ESTIMATED CALORIES BURNED 707

DIRECTIONS TO TRAILHEAD

From Route 6 in Provincetown, continue southwest to the highway's terminus at an intersection with Route 6A (signed for Provincetown), left, and Province Lands Road (signed for Race Point and Herring Cove Beach), right. Bear left on Route 6A. At 0.9 miles, where Route 6A veers left and becomes Bradford Street, you continue straight. Go another 0.2 miles to a rotary. There is roadside parking here on the right (curb) side of the rotary. Be sure to obey any NO PARKING signs. The trailhead is on the south side of the rotary, where a gap in a fence provides access to a dike across part of Provincetown Harbor.

Long Point

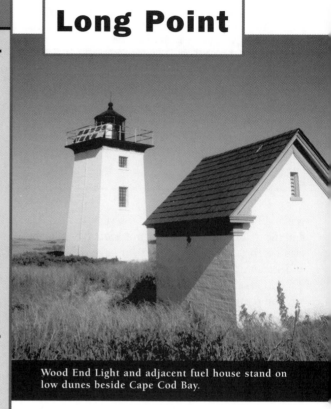

Wood End Light and adjacent fuel house stand on low dunes beside Cape Cod Bay.

WALK SUMMARY

This excursion, a fine off-season trek, takes you from the hustle and bustle of Provincetown, across Provincetown Harbor via a dike, to the remote, windswept tip of Cape Cod, where Long Point Light stands sentinel. Along the way, you'll also visit Wood End Light and stroll the sandy beach beside Cape Cod Bay. Bird-watching and plant study are just a few of the reasons to enjoy this walk, which should be reserved for a calm day. The dike and parts of the route are dangerous or impassible at high tide. Plan to start about two hours before low tide for Provincetown Harbor.

DESCRIPTION

Walk along the top of the mile-long dike, which is made of large boulders. Use caution on the uneven

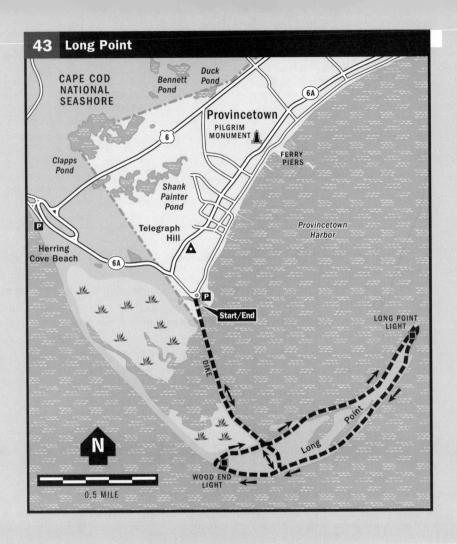

surface, especially if the boulders are wet. From the dike, you have fine views northeast of Provincetown Harbor and the Provincetown waterfront. Pilgrim Monument, a stone tower modeled after one in Siena, Italy, rises behind the buildings and wharves that front the harbor. To your right is a large salt marsh, with sand flats that are exposed as the tide drops. This is a good place to study gulls, terns, and shorebirds.

In the distance are two lighthouses—you'll visit both in a little while. To the left is Long Point Light, built in 1875 to replace an earlier structure dating from 1826. It stands just a few hundred yards from the very tip of Cape Cod. Ahead and slightly right is Wood End Light; the current structure dates from 1872, the year Congress approved creation of the U.S. Life Saving Service, a precursor of the Coast Guard.

FLORA	FAUNA
There is only one tree on this walk, a lone eastern red cedar, and it may soon be gone. There are plenty of other hardy plants however, including American beach grass, bayberry, salt-spray rose, dwarf sumac, seaside goldenrod, sea rocket, cocklebur, orach, beach pea, dusty miller, common saltwort, Virginia creeper, and poison ivy. In the salt marsh, look for salt hay, saltwater cordgrass, glasswort, sea lavender, and sea blite.	Gulls, terns, shorebirds, wading birds, and ducks all frequent this area. Look for the Cape's three common year-round gulls—great black-backed, herring, and ring billed—plus the three-season laughing gull. Of the shorebird tribe, likely candidates are greater yellowlegs, ruddy turnstone, red knot, black-bellied plover, sanderling, semipalmated sandpiper, semipalmated plover, and piping plover. Don't be surprised to see a northern harrier hunting over the low dunes.

After the dike meets the shore, it continues into low dunes that block your view of Cape Cod Bay. Clamber down the right side of the dike and follow a sandy path that meanders through the dunes, using caution around the plentiful poison ivy. Soon meet a multitude of paths, none of them official trails. Keep working your way south until you reach the shore of Cape Cod Bay. Turn right and go about 0.4 miles northwest along the beach. Watch carefully to find a path through low dunes to Wood End Light.

The lighthouse and its adjacent brick oil house are lonely but scenic sentinels on this deserted part of the Cape. To return to the dike, continue partway around the lighthouse to a path bordered by poison ivy that leads slightly east of north through the low dunes. After about 100 yards, reach the edge of the salt marsh. As you can see from the wrack line, the highest tides flood the marsh all the way to the dunes. Turn right and follow the shoreline to the dike. (To shorten the walk, follow the dike back to the parking area.)

When you reach the dike, at about the 2.2-mile point, cross it and head northeast, following the shoreline of Provincetown Harbor, which is to your left. Small patches of salt marsh, left, are exposed as the tide drops. Soon reach a broad channel that floods at high tide. Cross the channel (hopefully dry!) and continue along the beach, which may be soft sand or stones. Cross the next channel, which also floods at high tide.

Long Point Light sits on a low hill overlooking the tip of Cape Cod. A brick oil house is nearby, as is a white cross with the American flag. The flag and cross memorialize Charles S. Darby, who was killed in World War II. From the hill holding the cross, where poison ivy thrives, you'll have a great view of the lighthouse, Provincetown and its harbor, the Provincetown–Truro dunes, and Cape Cod Bay. On a clear day, you may be able to pick out the Wellfleet shoreline (southeast) and even Dennis, more than 18 miles to the south.

After stopping to admire the view, continue to follow the shoreline to the very tip of the Cape—a flat, gravelly sandbar, with clumps of beach grass clinging to slightly elevated hummocks. At about 3.7 miles, swing 180 degrees right around point of Long Point, and now head southwest along the shore of Cape Cod Bay. You may see sailboats, fishing boats, whale-watching boats, and even the passenger ferries that run between Boston and Provincetown's MacMillan Wharf.

In places, and depending on the tide, the beach narrows, bringing you close to the Bay's clear water and gently lapping waves. Low, grass-covered dunes soon block your view of Provincetown. Gulls and shorebirds may be plentiful along this part of the walk, roosting on sandbars exposed by the tide or feeding along the water's edge.

At about 5.3 miles, where the beach widens, look for a path heading right, through the dunes. As you follow this path, Pilgrim Monument should be ahead and slightly right. Where the path forks, stay left. At the next junction, where two trails join from the left, stay straight. Climb over a low rise and continue straight through the next junctions, following a broad, sandy path. The jumble of rocks ahead is actually the start of the dike. Your path skirts the dike on the left. Soon you close the loop at the edge of the salt marsh. From there, retrace your route across the dike to the parking area.

KEY AT-A-GLANCE INFORMATION

GENERAL

DISTANCE 6.6 miles

TYPE OF WALK Balloon

DIFFICULTY Difficult

TIME TO WALK 3–5 hours

MAPS *Cape Cod National Seashore*, National Geographic Maps; *Provincetown*, USGS

SCENERY Atlantic Ocean, Race Point Light, Hatches Harbor

EXPOSURE TO SUN Full

TRAIL TRAFFIC Heavy

TRAIL SURFACE(S) Dirt, pavement, sand

TRAILS OPEN All year

FEES/PASSES None

FACILITIES Restrooms, observation deck, phone; water, visitor center (both seasonal)

TRAIL USE

BICYCLES Allowed, but nearly 3 miles of route is on beach and sandy paths

DOGS Not allowed on bicycle trail, part of this route, May 1–October 31

HUNTING Not allowed

HEALTH STATS

NUMBER OF STEPS 14,850

ESTIMATED CALORIES BURNED 707

DIRECTIONS TO TRAILHEAD

From Route 6 in Provincetown, take Race Point Road northwest 1.4 miles; then turn right on the road to the Province Lands visitor center. Park in one of the several large, paved parking areas. The trailhead is on the north edge of the north parking area, just west of the visitor center.

Race Point and Hatches Harbor

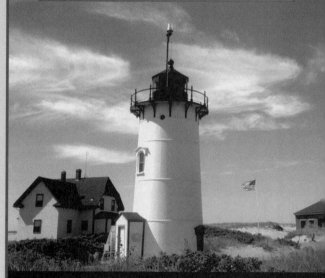

Race Point Light stands guard where the Atlantic Ocean meets Cape Cod Bay.

WALK SUMMARY

This walk in Cape Cod National Seashore takes you from the Province Lands Visitor Center to Race Point Light, on the westernmost tip of Provincetown. The route uses the paved Province Lands Bicycle Trail, the sandy Atlantic shoreline, and a dirt road atop a dike across Hatches Harbor, a beautiful salt mash. Start a few hours before the time of low tide for Race Point to find firm footing on the outer beach and to avoid flooded areas. This walk is best done off-season, on a day without wind.

DESCRIPTION

From the parking area, follow a paved path downhill, passing restrooms on your right and an amphitheater on your left. At a T-junction with the paved Province Lands Bicycle Trail, bear left. Staying on

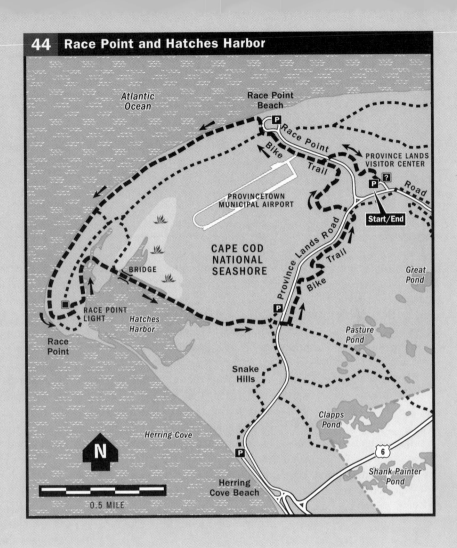

the right side of the bike trail, make a curvy but gentle descent through a stunted pitch-pine forest. In the hollows, or valleys, in the dunes, the pines are more sheltered from the wind, and hence grow taller.

Upon reaching Race Point Road, cross it carefully and walk a few more steps on the bike trail to a T-junction. Here turn right and follow a level stretch of the bike trail, parallel to Race Point Road. In the distance, off to the left, is Race Point Light, one of this walk's goals. Provincetown Municipal Airport is nearby, also on the left.

Cross over two roads to the airport, the first a service road, the second the main entrance. On a rolling course, soon reach a paved road, which is the start of the four-wheel-drive vehicle route to the outer beach. Cross the road,

FLORA	FAUNA
Pitch pine, Scotch pine, black oak, black cherry, eastern red cedar, and white poplar are among the trees found along this route. Bearberry, wild cranberry, poverty grass, and broom crowberry provide ground cover. Shrubs here include bayberry, highbush blueberry, black huckleberry, salt-spray rose, beach plum, sheep laurel, arrowwood, and groundsel tree. Goldenrods and asters provide color in late summer and fall, as do Virginia creeper and poison ivy.	In summer and fall, migrating shorebirds collect on the outer beach and in Hatches Harbor. Look for black-bellied plovers, greater yellowlegs, sanderlings, ruddy turnstones, whimbrels, and semipalmated sandpipers.

then continue on the bike trail for about 100 feet to where it ends at the lower parking area for Race Point Beach. Angle left and climb through this parking area for about 400 feet, toward the Race Point ranger station, a white building with a flagpole in front.

At the upper end of the parking area, follow the parking-area entrance road as it curves to the right; the ranger station should be on your left. After about 100 feet, nearing the west end of the upper parking area, bear left (northwest) on a sandy path north across the dunes. Race Point Beach and the Atlantic Ocean are directly ahead.

If you've timed your walk correctly, the tide should be on its way out, and you may be able to see the shallows and sandbars that spelled doom for many ships and mariners plying the coastal waters between Boston and New York. The wooden building in the distance to the right is the Old Harbor Life Saving Museum, built in 1897 and moved here from Chatham in 1977. The manned life-saving stations that once dotted the Cape's Atlantic shore provided the only hope of rescue from the ocean's icy waters when nor'easters pounded the coast with wind and surf.

Race Point Beach is a popular spot for sunbathing, swimming, and fishing. Vehicles with permits are allowed on the beach during limited times of the year; there are closures to protect nesting shorebirds, including piping plovers, which are federally listed as a threatened species. When you reach the beach, turn left and follow the shoreline southwest. The best footing is near the water's edge, on sand left damp by the receding tide. The vehicle track runs along the upper part of the beach; use caution when walking near it.

At about the 2.5-mile point, the vehicle track turns left and heads into the low dunes, but continue along the beach. You may notice that the water just offshore is rough. This is the "race," or current, where the Atlantic and Cape Cod Bay meet—hence the name Race Point, which is the westernmost part of Provincetown and site of Race Point Light. As you near the lighthouse, and before the beach makes a sharp bend to the left, look to your left: a path should be visible through the dunes. (If not, continue around the bend to a four-wheel-drive road; turn left on it to reach the lighthouse.)

Cut left through the dunes on soft sand, avoiding the border of poison ivy, and soon reach the lighthouse, the keeper's house, and several brick buildings. The smaller building, or oil house, was used to store fuel for the light; the larger building is the Race

Point Field Station. The first lighthouse here was built in 1816; the current lighthouse, keeper's house, and fuel house were built in 1876. With the lighthouse on your left, you meet the four-wheel-drive road (mentioned above) at a T-junction.

Turn left and then, almost immediately, veer right onto a sandy path. Follow a rolling course through low dunes, and then descend to a broad tidal channel that floods at high tide. Hug the left side of this channel, beside low dunes, for several hundred yards. At the point where the dunes end, turn right and cross the channel. (You should still have the lighthouse partially in view behind you.)

Once across, look for an obvious sandy draw heading northeast at an angle to the channel. A concrete marker with the inscription "Cable MMPWR" may be visible. Facing northeast into the draw, find a path angling right (southeast) through the dunes, which may be marked with a wooden post. As you crest a sandy rise, a dike and the vast expanse of Hatches Harbor, a 400-acre wetland, are visible ahead. Provincetown's Pilgrim Monument, modeled after a tower in Siena, Italy, rises in the distance.

Descend on the path to the dike, where you'll meet a dirt road. Follow the road across the dike, stopping to study the effects of a NPS restoration project, begun in 1987. Southwest of the dike is a salt marsh, one of nature's most fertile and productive ecosystems, which is flooded twice daily by the tide. The construction of the dike in 1930 cut off tidal flow to the area on the dike's northeast side. As a result, the marsh there suffered drastic changes, including a rise in invasive plant species, such as common reed, and an increase in mosquito larvae. The restoration project involves restoring the flow of saltwater to that area and has proved quite successful.

Continue on the road to about the 4.6-mile point, until you see the bike trail on your right. (This is just before you reach a small parking area adjacent to Province Lands Road.) Get on the bike trail by veering left, remembering to stay on its right side, and cross under Province Lands Road via a tunnel. About 100 feet ahead, the trail forks; here you bear left. Now comes the hilliest part of the route, as you roller-coaster up, over, and down the beautiful pine-studded dunes.

After a hairpin left turn, walk through a low tunnel (duck!) and then climb moderately to a junction, where you close the loop. From here, turn right, cross Race Point Road, and retrace your route to the parking area.

Martha's Vineyard

KEY AT-A-GLANCE INFORMATION

GENERAL

DISTANCE 1.6 miles

TYPE OF WALK Balloon

DIFFICULTY Moderate

TIME TO WALK 1–2 hours

MAPS *Fulling Mill Brook Preserve*, Martha's Vineyard Land Bank Commission; *Tisbury Great Pond*, USGS

SCENERY Forest

EXPOSURE TO SUN None

TRAIL TRAFFIC Light

TRAIL SURFACE(S) Dirt

TRAILS OPEN All year

FEES/PASSES None

FACILITIES None

TRAIL USE

BICYCLES Allowed

DOGS Allowed on leash April 15–August 31; leashed or under voice control September 1–April 14

HUNTING This preserve is closed to the public during deer shotgun week, generally the first week in December.

HEALTH STATS

NUMBER OF STEPS 3,600

ESTIMATED CALORIES BURNED 171

DIRECTIONS TO TRAILHEAD

From the intersection of Middle and Tabor House roads in Chilmark, take Middle Road southwest 0.5 miles to Henry Hough Lane and turn left. Go about 100 feet to a dirt road, turn left, and go several hundred feet to a dirt parking area. The trailhead is on the east corner of the parking area.

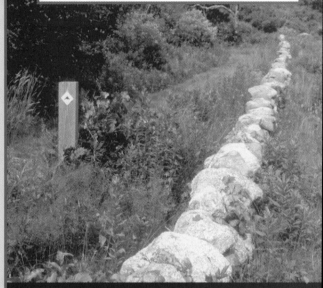

Stone walls remind visitors of the island's agricultural heritage.

Fulling Mill Brook

WALK SUMMARY

Five distinct plant communities are found on this 50-acre preserve: mesic (moist) hardwood forest, successional shrubland, red-maple swamp, mixed-oak woodland, and herbaceous grassland. Sample them all on this sometimes-hilly excursion, which traces the length of Fulling Mill Brook between Middle and South roads. The term *fulling* refers to a process whereby fabric is cleaned and pre-shrunk before being made into clothing. This process was carried out by early settlers in a water-powered mill; the source of water was called a fulling-mill brook.

DESCRIPTION

The Green Trail, unsigned, descends from the parking area through an oak woodland to a tributary of

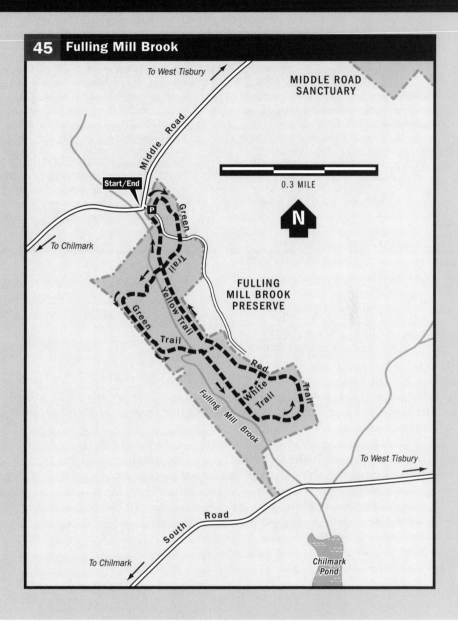

45 **Fulling Mill Brook**

Fulling Mill Brook, which you cross via a bridge. Now climb a wide dirt trail, cross Henry Hough Lane, and continue on the trail. Henry Beetle Hough was editor of the *Vineyard Gazette*, the island's newspaper, from 1920 until 1968. Descend to cross another dirt road, shown on the map as the Yellow Trail but signed with a blue marker. Beyond the road, a bridge takes you across Fulling Mill Brook.

Climb away from the brook, passing large glacial boulders, and soon reach a rocky ridgetop. Rock walls are common on Martha's Vineyard—this route takes you beside some and through gaps in others. Now the trail winds moderately downhill to a boardwalk with a rest bench in a red-maple swamp. Wooden steps lead downhill to Fulling Mill Brook, which you cross on a bridge.

With the creek now on your right, cross a rock bridge over Fulling Mill Brook and soon reach a T-junction (shown on the map as a four-way) with the Yellow Trail, which here is a dirt road signed with a blue marker. Turn right and enjoy a level stroll, soon passing the White Trail on your left. A large, picturesque meadow is left. At the meadow's south end, turn left on the Red Trail (the Yellow Trail continues south from here to a trailhead on South Road).

With the meadow now left and a wooded area on your right, curve left and climb to a junction with the White Trail, left. Continue straight, pass through a gap in a stone wall, and again merge with the Yellow Trail (signed blue). At the next junction, a four-way, stay on the Yellow Trail by going straight. Soon meet Henry Hough Lane at a T-junction. Turn left and follow the dirt road (used by vehicles) about 100 yards or so to the parking-area entrance road. Turn right and go several hundred feet to the parking area.

Rock and Roll

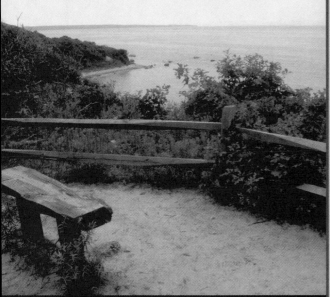

View westward from Blue Trail overlook takes in Vineyard Sound and Great Rock Bight.

WALK SUMMARY

At just under 30 acres, this preserve boasts three distinct plant communities: black-oak woodland, mesic (damp) woodland, and coastal bank and dune. Also here is a stop along the African American Heritage Trail of Martha's Vineyard, marked by a rock with a commemorative plaque. The preserve's namesake rock sits just offshore in a cove, or bight, on Vineyard Sound and is visible from an overlook atop a coastal cliff. A network of short, easy trails connects these various points of interest; one trail loops most of the way around Marl Pond, a red maple–tupelo swamp.

DESCRIPTION

Two trails depart from the trailhead, which has an information board and a map—Blue going straight

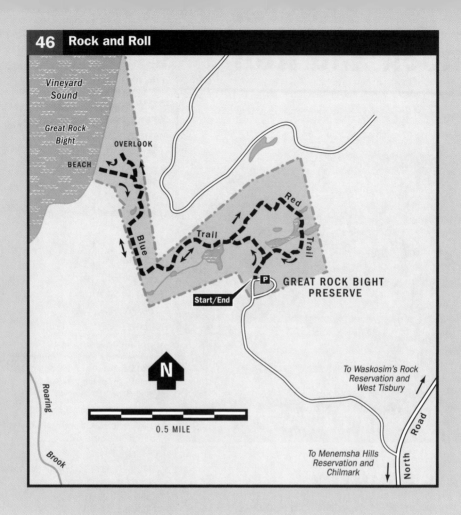

Vineyard
Sound

Great Rock
Bight

OVERLOOK

BEACH

Red
Trail

Blue

Trail

Red
Trail

P GREAT ROCK BIGHT
PRESERVE

Start/End

N

0.5 MILE

To Waskosim's Rock
Reservation and
West Tisbury

Roaring

Brook

To Menemsha Hills
Reservation and
Chilmark

North
Road

(northeast), Yellow to the left (northwest). Take the Blue Trail, a gravelly dirt path that curves left and soon passes the Red Trail, right, which forms part of the Marl Pond Loop. Now curve left and cross a bridge over a seasonal stream. A level walk leads to another junction with the Red Trail to your right.

Go straight, toward the beach, and enjoy a rolling ramble through relatively open, parklike terrain, with a pond on the left. At the next junction, where the Yellow Trail joins from the left, turn right to stay on the Blue Trail. From here to the beach, bicycles and horses are prohibited, and a narrow gap in a fence prevents their passage.

A nearby rock with a metal plaque, part of the African American Heritage Trail of Martha's Vineyard, commemorates Rebecca, an African woman enslaved in Chilmark who later became free and inherited substantial property on Martha's Vineyard, including this land.

The Blue Trail descends—gently, then moderately—beside a stone wall, passing a rest bench, which is to the right. Soon turn right and cross a small stream via a wooden bridge. Another rest bench sits to your right, and Vineyard Sound is visible to the left through a screen of trees. Clamber down a steep pitch, aided by dirt steps. At a junction just ahead, a short trail goes straight to a viewpoint with a rest bench. From here, the vista extends across Great Rock Bight, with its namesake rock, westward to the Elizabeth Islands.

To reach the beach, return to the previous junction and bear sharply right. Follow the rocky, eroded trail steeply downhill to a narrow strand of sandy shore. When ready, retrace your route to a junction with the Red Trail (the first of two), at about the 1-mile point. Turn left, then curve right and climb a low rise. There is a rest bench on the right. Now wind almost imperceptibly downhill to Marl Pond, which sits amid a red maple–tupelo swamp.

Cross wet areas via a boardwalk and enjoy the rich, almost junglelike vegetation, so different from the scrubby growth found at the beach. The island's largest stand of hop hornbeam—tall, tough-wooded trees with soft, doubly serrated leaves—is nearby. After passing a rest bench, right, rejoin the Blue Trail, turn left, and retrace your route a few hundred feet to the parking area.

KEY AT-A-GLANCE INFORMATION

GENERAL

DISTANCE 3.8 miles

TYPE OF WALK Balloon

DIFFICULTY Moderate

TIME TO WALK 2–3 hours

MAPS *Menemsha Hills*, The Trustees of Reservations; *Tisbury Great Pond*, USGS

SCENERY Forest, Vineyard Sound

EXPOSURE TO SUN Partial

TRAIL TRAFFIC Moderate

TRAIL SURFACE(S) Dirt

TRAILS OPEN All year

FEES/PASSES Voluntary donation

FACILITIES Toilet (seasonal)

TRAIL USE

BICYCLES Not allowed

DOGS Not allowed

HUNTING Not allowed

HEALTH STATS

NUMBER OF STEPS 8,550

ESTIMATED CALORIES BURNED 407

DIRECTIONS TO TRAILHEAD

From the intersection of North and Tabor House roads in Chilmark, take North Road southwest for 0.7 miles, turn right, and go 0.1 mile to a small dirt parking area, right. The trailhead is on the west corner of the parking area.

A Hill Too High

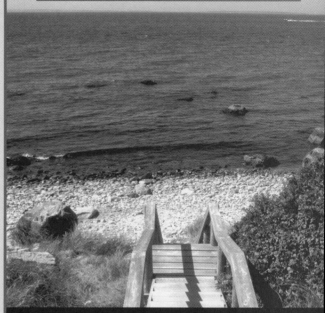

Steps aid final descent to beach on Vineyard Sound.

WALK SUMMARY

Two scenic vantage points, one atop Prospect Hill and the other overlooking Vineyard Sound, draw visitors to this 211-acre beachfront reserve, a mostly forested realm of tall oaks and colorful-in-fall tupelos. The route consists of two loops, linked by short out-and-back trail segments.

DESCRIPTION

From the trailhead, follow a dirt and sometimes-muddy trail past an information board, which has a small map of the reservation. A glacial moraine forms the elevated spine of Martha's Vineyard, and evidence of this icy past—rocks and boulders—is nearby. Stay left at a fork signed for the Harris Loop to Prospect Hill and the Great Sand Bank (signed elsewhere as Great Sand Cliff). The root-crossed

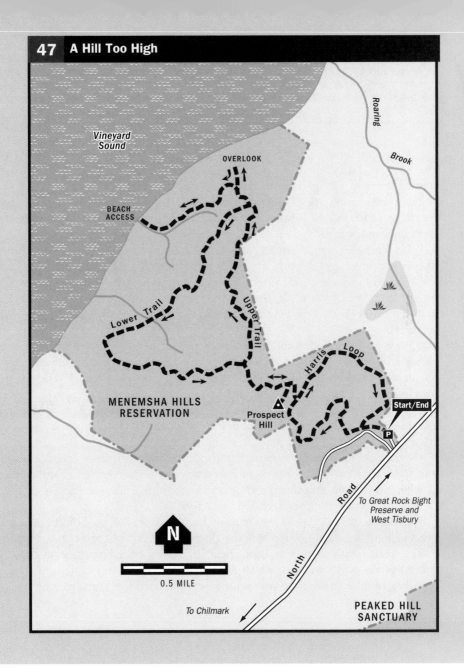

trail soon begins to climb gently toward Prospect Hill. At 308 feet, this was the second highest point on Martha's Vineyard, but supposedly some competitive folks made it the highest by piling rocks on the summit. (Or perhaps that's a tall tale spun for gullible tourists and guidebook authors.)

> **FLORA**
>
> A rich array of trees and shrubs—among them black oak, white oak, scrub oak, black cherry, red maple, American beech, sassafras, tupelo, sweet pepperbush, bayberry, highbush blueberry, arrowwood, and black huckleberry—will delight plant enthusiasts.

At the next junction, leave the Harris Loop by turning left on the single-track Upper Trail. After several hundred feet, turn left again on the trail to Prospect Hill, which is crowned by a large pile of boulders. The view from the summit, although blocked to the north and east by tall oaks, is splendid, taking in Menemsha Pond, the coastal curve of Menemsha Bight, and the lighthouse at Gay Head. When ready, retrace your route to the Upper Trail and bear left.

Descend over rough ground, passing a handful of magnificent, venerable white oaks. Continue straight through a four-way junction with a dirt road, and then reach a fork. Veer right to stay on the Upper Trail—the left branch is the Lower Trail, which you will use later. Level for a while, the trail now begins a curvy, rolling course that leads through more open, shrubby terrain, where stone walls lie partially buried under boughs and brambles.

Soon the other end of the Lower Trail joins on the left; you will return here in a few minutes. For now, however, follow the Upper Trail to the next junction and then go straight on a short boardwalk to the Great Sand Cliff overlook, where 360-degree views await, including a magnificent panorama of Vineyard Sound. After enjoying the scene, return to the Upper Trail and turn right. The trail, which also has sections of boardwalk, descends, sometimes steeply via steps, to a rocky beach. When ready, retrace your route on the Upper Trail to the near junction with the Lower Trail.

Turn right on a single-track trail and descend through dense forest, crossing a sometimes-wet area on a boardwalk and then wooden planks. Regain a shrubbier habitat, where wild grape, greenbrier, and poison ivy form impenetrable thickets. The landscape may be gentle, but the vegetation certainly isn't!

Passing a stand of tupelo trees in a low-lying area, the trail now climbs moderately over rough ground. At a junction with the Upper Trail, bear right and retrace your route to the junction with the Harris Loop. Bear left, following red markers on trees, and descend gently past a wetland, which is to your left. Now gain elevation to close the loop; then turn left and retrace your route several hundred feet to the parking area.

Hillside Overlook

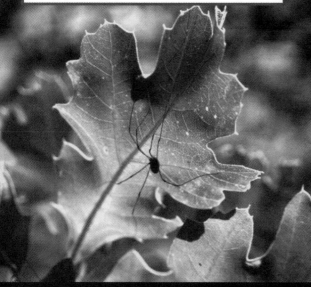

The heavily wooded Middle Road Sanctuary is a great place to study local flora and fauna.

 KEY AT-A-GLANCE INFORMATION

GENERAL

DISTANCE 2.2 miles

TYPE OF WALK Balloon

DIFFICULTY Moderate

TIME TO WALK 1–2 hours

MAPS *Tisbury Great Pond*, USGS

SCENERY Forest

EXPOSURE TO SUN Partial

TRAIL TRAFFIC Light

TRAIL SURFACE(S) Dirt

TRAILS OPEN All year

FEES/PASSES None

FACILITIES None

TRAIL USE

BICYCLES Trails not suitable for bicycles

DOGS Allowed on leash

HUNTING Not allowed

HEALTH STATS

NUMBER OF STEPS 4,950

ESTIMATED CALORIES BURNED 236

DIRECTIONS TO TRAILHEAD

From the intersection of Middle and Meetinghouse roads in Chilmark, take Middle Road southwest 0.4 miles to a very small parking area on your left. The trailhead is on the south side of the parking area.

WALK SUMMARY

This route explores a hilly, forested sanctuary, owned by the Sheriff's Meadow Foundation and located just off Middle Road in Chilmark. The destination is an overlook on a steep southeast-facing hillside, where there are views of the Vineyard's Atlantic coast and a rest bench.

DESCRIPTION

From the trailhead, where there is a board with a sketch map of the sanctuary, follow the single-track Red Trail (unsigned) into a mostly white-oak woodland. Martha's Vineyard, like Cape Cod and Nantucket, is home to the ticks that transmit Lyme disease. A device located just beyond the trailhead and off the trail uses corn to attract deer, which are the tick's primary hosts. When the deer try to

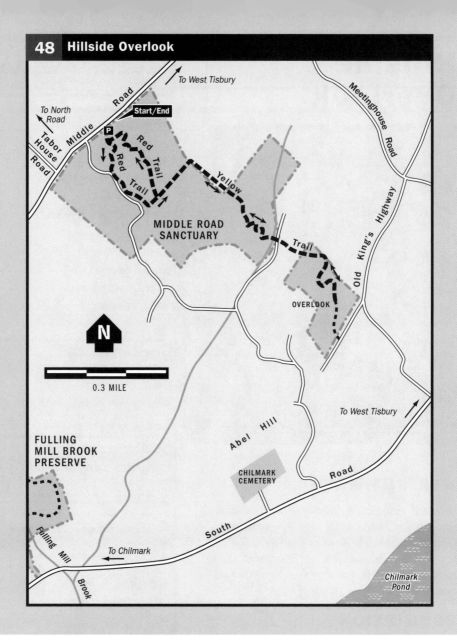

To West Tisbury

To North Road

Start/End

Middle Road

Tabor House Road

Red Trail

Red Trail

Yellow

MIDDLE ROAD SANCTUARY

Trail

Meetinghouse Road

Old King's Highway

OVERLOOK

N

0.3 MILE

FULLING MILL BROOK PRESERVE

To West Tisbury

Abel Hill

CHILMARK CEMETERY

Road

South

Fulling Mill

To Chilmark

Brook

Chilmark Pond

eat the corn, they must first brush against material saturated with Permethrin, a tick repellent. Hopefully, this device and others like it will help control the spread of Lyme disease.

A curvy course leads to a junction marked by a trail post. Stay on the Red Trail by turning right; then climb on a gentle grade. At a T-junction, turn left on

FLORA	FAUNA
The forest here features white oak, black oak, shadbush, American beech, sassafras, and black cherry, with an understory of shrubs such as highbush blueberry, lowbush blueberry, black huckleberry, hazelnut, scrub oak, dwarf sumac, and wild raisin.	The dense vegetation may make birds hard to see, but you can practice identifying blue jays, eastern towhees, and other songbirds by their calls. Various species of raptors, including red-tailed hawks and osprey, also make distinctive sounds, usually high-pitched cries.

a well-trodden path, still the Red Trail, and continue climbing. Crest a low rise and descend to a junction not shown on the sketch map at the trailhead. Turn left to stay on the Red Trail (the trail going straight leads to the sanctuary boundary).

At the next junction, the Red Trail goes left back to the parking area, and the Yellow Trail goes straight. Follow the Yellow Trail into a sandier, more open habitat dotted with a few glacial boulders. After rising gently for a while, the trail curves right and descends through dense forest. Ahead, where a faint path angles left, an arrow directs you right. The ensuing slalom course drops gently to a four-way junction with a dirt road.

Cross the road and climb on a gentle, then moderate, grade, passing a few homes on the way. Go through a gap in a stone wall and then reach level ground, where an arrow directs you left at a junction. Descend through a narrow corridor of shrubs to a rest bench on your right. By standing on the bench, you'll have a limited view southeast toward Chilmark Pond and the Vineyard's Atlantic coast. When ready, retrace your route to the junction of the Yellow and Red trails.

Turn right on the Red Trail and enjoy a gentle downhill ramble through a shady forest, passing more glacial boulders. Now the trail winds moderately downhill to close the Red Trail loop. From here, bear slightly right and retrace your route to the parking area.

KEY AT-A-GLANCE INFORMATION

GENERAL

DISTANCE 1.3 miles

TYPE OF WALK Loop

DIFFICULTY Moderate

TIME TO WALK 1 hour or less

MAPS *Peaked Hill Reservation,* Martha's Vineyard Land Bank Commission; *Tisbury Great Pond,* USGS

SCENERY Forest, meadow

EXPOSURE TO SUN Partial

TRAIL TRAFFIC Light

TRAIL SURFACE(S) Dirt

TRAILS OPEN All year

FEES/PASSES None

FACILITIES None

TRAIL USE

BICYCLES Allowed

DOGS Allowed on leash or under voice control

HUNTING General hunting in season is allowed on this preserve, which is closed to the public during deer shotgun week, generally the first week in December; hunting is prohibited on Sunday and Monday, except during deer shotgun week, when hunting does occur on Monday.

HEALTH STATS

NUMBER OF STEPS 2,925

ESTIMATED CALORIES BURNED 139

DIRECTIONS TO TRAILHEAD

From the intersection of Middle and Tabor House roads in Chilmark, take Tabor House Road northwest 0.5 miles and turn left onto unsigned Pasture Road, an unimproved dirt road. Stay right at the next 2 intersections, following Land Bank signs. At 0.8 miles, there is a small dirt parking area. The trailhead is on the southwest side of the parking area.

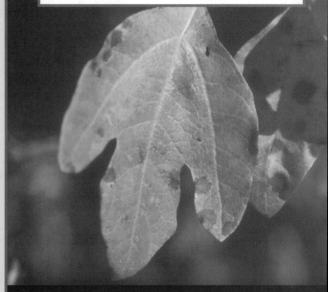

Sassafras is a tree with oddly shaped leaves, sometimes described as looking like mittens.

WALK SUMMARY

This 132.5-acre reservation, consisting mostly of mixed-oak woodland, meadow and pasture, and greenbrier thickets, is home to about 170 plant species and 50 bird species. The route climbs to several high points, where views may be limited by fast-growing trees and shrubs, but doesn't reach the summit of 311-foot Peaked Hill, the island's highest point. *Note:* Trail names (colors) on the latest Land Bank map may not correspond in all cases to signage or to names on older maps.

DESCRIPTION

Two trails, Blue and Yellow, depart from this parking area. Take the Blue Trail southwest from the trailhead, passing an information board and a trail-map box. Glacial boulders line the level trail, which

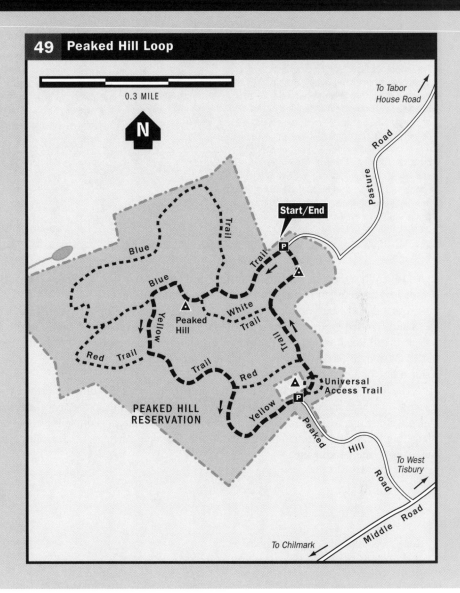

To Tabor
House Road

0.3 MILE

N

Start/End

PEAKED HILL
RESERVATION

Peaked
Hill

Universal
Access Trail

To West
Tisbury

To Chilmark

Middle Road

soon reaches a junction. Bear left, still on the Blue Trail, and climb past the White Trail, which goes left. In a clearing, ahead, there are some limited views to the north. Peaked Hill—at 311 feet the island's official highest point—is southeast, behind a screen of trees and shrubs.

At a fork, bear left onto the Yellow Trail and descend gently through an oak forest. On a breezy day, the rustling oak leaves create a sonorous serenade, punctuated perhaps by a mournful note from an offshore buoy. Reaching a low point beside a huge, overgrown meadow on your right, the trail curves left and

FLORA

The mixed-oak woodland here consists mainly of white oak, black oak, pitch pine, tupelo, and hickory. Other trees on the reservation include red maple, black cherry, and sassafras. Shrubs such as arrowwood, black huckleberry, highbush blueberry, hazelnut, scrub oak, dwarf sumac, sweet pepperbush, and bayberry line the route. Ferns and vines—greenbrier, poison ivy, wild rose, wild grape, Virginia creeper, and blackberry—form junglelike thickets. Colorful wildflowers bloom in the reservation's open areas, especially near the meadow.

FAUNA

Common woodland birds here include blue jay, gray catbird, song sparrow, black-capped chickadee, white-breasted nuthatch, Carolina wren, and various warblers.

begins to climb on a gentle grade. Bear right at a fork to stay on the Yellow Trail, which threads its way between the oak forest, left, and the meadow.

The trail now curves left and enters the forest, winding uphill via tight S-bends over sandy, eroded ground. Soon reach Radar Hill, a commanding viewpoint at the end of Peaked Hill Road, which was the site of a military lookout and garrison during World War II. Bear right, cross the paved road, and then find a dirt road heading northeast, beside a line of autumn olive trees.

The road ends after several hundred feet, but a trail continues northeast and descends gently to a four-way junction with a dirt road, shown on the map as the Red Trail. Go straight across the road and follow a rolling, meandering course through forest. A large boulder marks a junction with the White Trail, left. Angle right and enjoy a level walk back to the parking area.

Waskosim's Rock

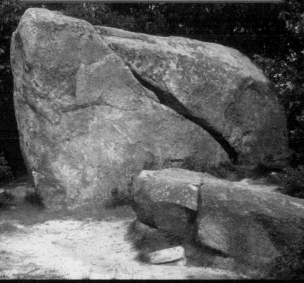

Waskosim's Rock was used in colonial times as a benchmark to divide British and Wampanoag lands.

WALK SUMMARY

This reservation is named for a huge glacial boulder that once served as a benchmark for establishing the boundary between lands of the native Wampanoags and property claimed by English settlers. Many trails, generally in the form of three loops, crisscross the hilly terrain, which is divided between woodland and meadow. *Note:* Trail names (colors) on the latest Land Bank map may not correspond in all cases to signage or to names on older maps.

DESCRIPTION

From the trailhead, where there is an information board with a sketch map, take the wide and level Blue Trail into a dense woodland with a rain-forest feel. Cross Mill Brook on a bridge; then come to a four-way junction. Here the Blue Trail goes straight

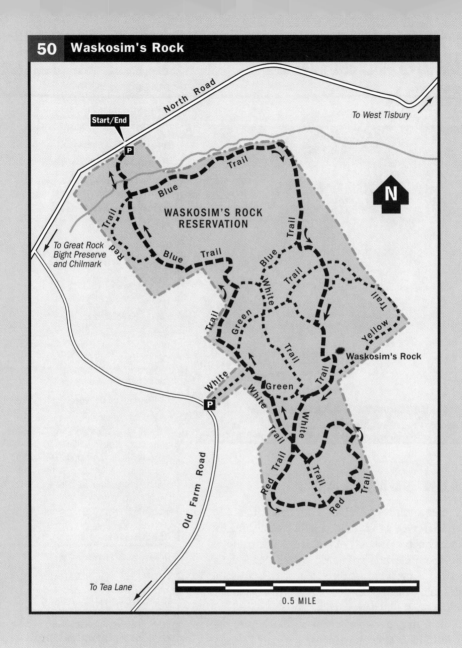

To West Tisbury

Start/End

North Road

WASKOSIM'S ROCK RESERVATION

N

Blue Trail

To Great Rock Bight Preserve and Chilmark

Blue Trail

Red Trail

Trail

Blue Trail

White Trail

Green Trail

Trail

Yellow Trail

Waskosim's Rock

White Trail

Green

White Trail

Old Farm Road

Red Trail

White Trail

Red Trail

To Tea Lane

0.5 MILE

and left; the Red Trail goes right. Turn left and traverse a possibly wet area on split logs. Cross a stone wall via steps and wander beside Mill Brook, which is left. On a sunny day, light dazzles from the broad, flat leaves of American beech trees. Large rocks and boulders recall the island's glacial past.

Now the trail curves right and traces a line between forest on your right and an overgrown meadow to your left. Where the Blue Trail goes right, switch to the Green Trail by bearing left. After another 0.1 mile or so, angle right at a fork and, in about 50 feet, come to a four-way junction, where the Yellow Trail departs to the left. Go straight, still on the Green Trail, and climb gently, then moderately, through a wooded area that soon gives way to shrubland.

The trail snakes its way uphill to a junction with the joined Green and Yellow trails on the left, at about the 1-mile point. Bear right and continue climbing, now over open sandy ground, to a T-junction (shown incorrectly on the map). Bear left and descend slightly to Waskosim's Rock, a huge glacial boulder split diagonally almost in half. The rock is some 50 or 60 feet in circumference. In Colonial times, it was used as a bench-mark for a line between here and Menemsha Pond, which divided British from Wampanoag lands. Today the rock sits astride the Chilmark–West Tisbury town line.

Continue straight past the rock, which is on your left. Where the Yellow Trail joins sharply from the left, bear right to stay on the Green Trail. Descend gently and curve right to a junction (shown incorrectly as a wide fork on the map) with the White Trail, near a gap in a stone wall. Turn left, keep the wall on your right, and go about 100 yards to meet the Red Trail, which joins from the right via a stile. At an upcoming fork, bear right on the Red Trail, a narrow track in dense forest. Continue straight through a four-way junction, where the White Trail goes left and an unofficial trail goes right.

Now the trail curves left beside a stone wall and meets the White Trail, which merges on the left. Bear right and soon close the Red Trail loop. Now retrace your route to the next junction, where the Red Trail goes left and climbs via steps over a stone wall. Turn left, cross the wall, and climb gently to meet the Green Trail. Go left, climb over a rise, and then follow a rolling course to an obscure junction (shown incorrectly on the map), which is on a pine-fringed hilltop overlooking a large meadow.

Turn right to stay on the Green Trail; then descend into forest, with a stone wall on your left. Go straight at the next junction, now on the White Trail, and cross a creek via a plank bridge. Meet a dirt road at a T-junction, where an elderly/handicapped parking area is just left. Turn right and follow the White Trail between dense forest and an open field.

Soon turn left onto the Blue Trail, wander through a narrow corridor of shrubs and vines, and then curve left to climb a ridge. Follow a level course beside a stone wall on your right and then descend to a junction with the Red Trail, which departs left. Con-tinue straight to a four-way junction, which closes the Blue Trail loop. From here, go straight and retrace your route to the parking area.

GENERAL

DISTANCE 2.5 miles

TYPE OF WALK Double loop with short string between

DIFFICULTY Moderate

TIME TO WALK 1–2 hours

MAPS *Vineyard Haven*, USGS

SCENERY Pond, forest, Vineyard Sound, wetland

EXPOSURE TO SUN Partial

TRAIL TRAFFIC Moderate

TRAIL SURFACE(S) Dirt, sand

TRAILS OPEN All year

FEES/PASSES None

FACILITIES Information kiosk, staffed on summer weekends

TRAIL USE

BICYCLES Not allowed

DOGS Allowed on leash

HUNTING Not allowed

HEALTH STATS

NUMBER OF STEPS 5,625

ESTIMATED CALORIES BURNED 268

DIRECTIONS TO TRAILHEAD

From the intersection of State and South Indian Hill roads in West Tisbury, take South Indian Hill Road northwest for 0.3 miles to an intersection with a stop sign. Turn left on Indian Hill Road, go 1.3 miles to Obed Daggett Road, and turn right. The road, paved at first, soon becomes dirt. Dirt driveways diverge from the dirt road, but SANCTUARY signs help you keep on track. At 1.1 mile there is a dirt parking area, which serves two trailheads. The trailhead for this walk is on the south side of the parking area.

Beach, Pond, and Forest

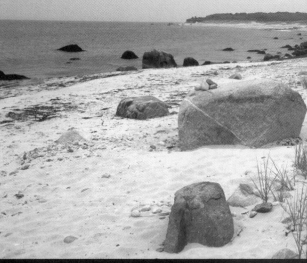

The Vineyard Sound beach is studded with glacial boulders.

WALK SUMMARY

With more than 300 prime acres, this sanctuary, preserved by the Sheriff's Meadow Foundation, offers visitors the chance to explore beach, forest, and wetland habitats and to revel in views of Vineyard Sound and the Elizabeth Islands from atop a seaside overlook. There is a rich history of land preservation here as well. One of the cofounders of the Sheriff's Meadow Foundation, a local land trust, was Henry Beetle Hough, award-winning editor of the *Vineyard Gazette*, the island's newspaper. The Hough homestead is nearby, and the Hough family donated 70 acres to help create the sanctuary. The Daggett family, long-time residents, sold the foundation 100 acres at a price well below market value to protect the area's fragile beauty. The

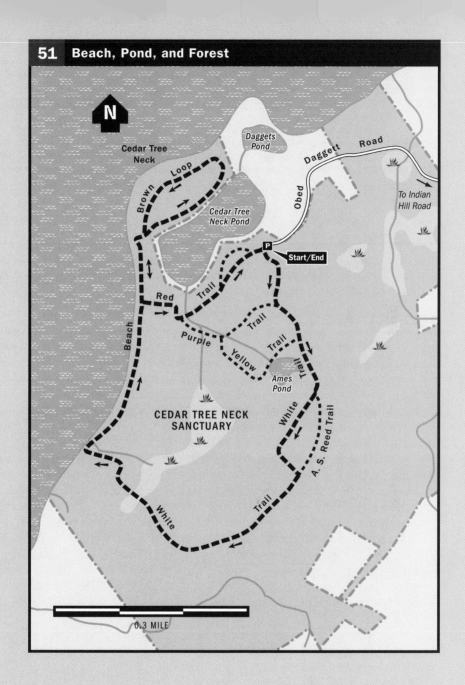

FLORA	FAUNA
Because of the many habitats, this is a rich area for plant study. Trees include American beech, red pine, black oak, white oak, red maple, tupelo, sassafras, sumac, and eastern red cedar. Forming the forest understory are arrowwood, bayberry, sweet pepperbush, and swamp azalea, along with poison ivy, green-brier, Virginia creeper, and various ferns. Dune plants include American beach grass, cockle-bur, orach, common saltwort, beach pea, and salt-spray rose. Grape vines, roses, and wild-flowers grace the Brown Trail.	Great black-backed gulls, terns, and double-crested cormorants may be visible from the beach. In the dense woodlands, songs and calls are often the best way to identify birds. Listen for the prairie warbler's rapidly ascending whistle, the common yellowthroat's "witchity, witchity, witchity, witch," and the song sparrow's musical phrase, which usually starts with three distinct notes.

Foundation purchased another 40 acres through a gift from the family of Alexander S. Reed, an avid birder and naturalist.

DESCRIPTION

At the trailhead, there is an information kiosk with maps and information about native plants. Take the White Trail, a sandy path, and walk south through a dense, shady woodland, climbing on a gentle grade. The White Trail here is part of the Bruce Irons Trail, dedicated to R. Bruce Irons III, a North Carolina educator who frequently visited Martha's Vineyard with his family. When Irons died of cancer in 1988—he was only 46 years old—his wife and children honored him through a gift to support land conservation on the island.

Pass the Purple Trail, which goes right, and enter a forest of red pine, many of them dying and riddled with woodpecker holes. Where the Yellow/Bruce Irons Trail goes right, continue straight, with the air perhaps fragrant from swamp azalea, which blooms in early summer. Soon pass the A. S. Reed Trail, on the left, which connects with the Alexander S. Reed Bird Refuge. Several more trails, unofficial, depart from the described route.

Climb a leaf-carpeted trail to gain a ridgetop; then descend gently and curve right. Cross a tupelo–red maple swamp via a boardwalk; then follow a rolling course that soon winds downhill through a narrow, shrubby corridor to a beach on Vineyard Sound, where waves may be gently lapping the rock-strewn shore. Across Vineyard Sound lie the Elizabeth Islands, which run southwest from Woods Hole on Cape Cod and border Buzzards Bay.

Turn right and enjoy a seaside stroll amid glacial boulders. After about 0.3 miles, pass a trail leading right, through a low dune. (To shorten the walk, turn right here and follow the description below.) Go another 0.1 mile or so; then turn right and climb a set of steps leading away from the beach. Now on the Brown Trail, there is a fine view of Cedar Tree Neck Pond, ahead and right.

Where the Brown Trail forks to begin a loop, stay right. Vine tendrils reach out to touch you in a narrow corridor, then a tunnel, of shrubs and wind-pruned trees. Leaves rustling in the wind may add to the eerie feeling. The trail curves left and climbs, regaining seaward views. For an even better vista, climb a short trail, right, to a bluff with a rest bench. This headland overlooks Vineyard Sound and Elizabeth Islands.

Descend from this airy perch, turn right, and soon close the loop. Now turn right again and retrace your route to the beach. Turn left and retrace your route on the beach for about 0.1 mile, to where a trail goes left through a low dune. Turn left and soon gain higher ground, with Cedar Tree Neck Pond on the left. The trail here is a sandy path bordered by ropes strung through poles. At an impenetrable thicket of scrub, the trail veers right.

Cross the creek joining Cedar Tree Neck and Ames ponds; then climb to a junction. Turn sharply left on the Red Trail and climb past a stand of marvelously twisted, drooping American beech trees, where a sign urges visitors not to carve into the bark of living trees. The route crests a rise, then descends past two unofficial trails, both left. Where the Red Trail splits, stay straight, cross a creek via a plank bridge, and then climb to the parking area.

Sandplain Sortie

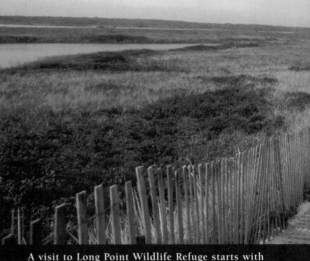

A visit to Long Point Wildlife Refuge starts with a walk to a popular swimming beach.

WALK SUMMARY

Don't miss this stimulating walk, which traverses a popular Atlantic Ocean beach and then seeks solitude in a wildlife refuge graced with a variety of habitats and plant communities, all managed by The Trustees of Reservations, a Massachusetts land-conservation organization founded in 1891. Guided canoe and kayak tours of adjacent Tisbury Great Pond are offered by The Trustees, (508) 693-7392. *Note:* The summer parking area may fill early in the day; please have an alternate destination in mind.

DESCRIPTION

From the trailhead, pass an information board and walk on either of two parallel dirt roads that head southwest toward the barrier beach. After about 100 yards, the roads join at a handicapped-parking

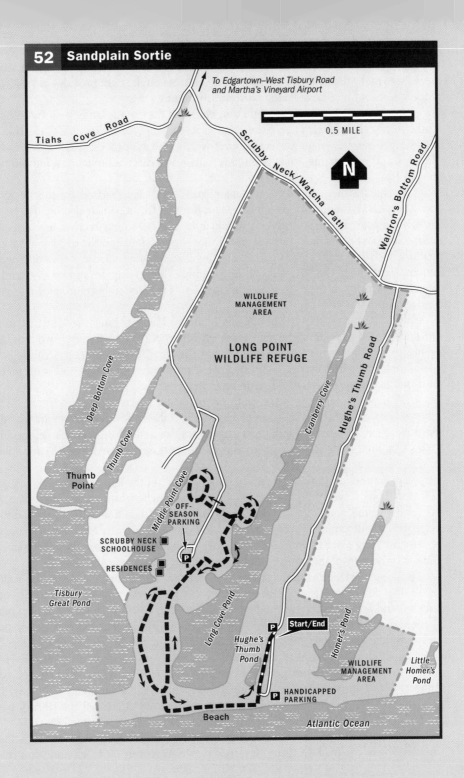

To Edgartown–West Tisbury Road
and Martha's Vineyard Airport

0.5 MILE

N

Tiahs Cove Road

Scrubby Neck/Watcha Path

Waldron's Bottom Road

WILDLIFE
MANAGEMENT
AREA

**LONG POINT
WILDLIFE REFUGE**

Deep Bottom Cove

Thumb Cove

Cranberry Cove

Hughe's Thumb Road

Thumb
Point

Middle Point Cove

OFF-
SEASON
PARKING

SCRUBBY NECK
SCHOOLHOUSE

RESIDENCES

Tisbury
Great Pond

Long Cove Pond

P

Start/End

Hughe's
Thumb
Pond

Homer's Pond

WILDLIFE
MANAGEMENT
AREA

Little
Homer's
Pond

P HANDICAPPED
PARKING

Beach

Atlantic Ocean

203

area just southeast of Hughe's Thumb Pond. Now cross a low dune via a boardwalk and gain the outer beach. Turn right and take a seaside stroll along a sandy strand, with the wave-tossed Atlantic Ocean to your left. A clearing on the right provides access to the gentle waters of Long Cove Pond, a favorite swimming spot.

After about 0.5 miles, turn right and cross the dune on a sandy path (please stay off the dunes elsewhere). Long Cove Pond is to your right, and Tisbury Great Pond, a much larger body of water perhaps dotted with sailboats, canoes, and kayaks, is left. After descending from the dune, continue straight on a dirt road, passing a mowed path on your left.

The habitat here is called sandplain grassland, characterized by mostly open, grassy terrain. The sandplain communities on the East Coast, which also include heathlands, pine barrens, and scrub-oak shrublands, are becoming increasingly rare and threatened ecosystems due to development, fire suppression, and the decline of agricultural use such as grazing, mowing, and clearing. Land-management agencies and organizations, including The Trustees of Reservations, are trying to preserve sandplain communities through the use of such techniques as prescribed burning, mowing, grazing, and cutting.

About 0.4 miles from the beach, you'll reach a four-way junction—the road going straight is closed to visitors; the road going left is part of the return route. Two buildings are nearby: the larger is a staff residence, and the smaller is the former Scrubby Neck Schoolhouse, which closed in 1889. Bear right on a grassy dirt road and soon meet a short trail that goes left to the off-season parking area.

(*Off-season parking area start:* From the trailhead, which is on the southwest side, follow a mowed path beside a maintenance shed about 150 feet to an information board. Bear left, go several hundred feet to the edge of a meadow, and bear left again at a fork. Continue straight to the grassy dirt road mentioned above, turn left, and follow the description below.)

Pass another trail to the off-season parking area, on the left, and now enjoy a level walk near Long Cove Pond, which is right. Soon branch right on a trail that wanders even closer to the pond. Now rejoin the dirt road at a T-junction, turn right, and then merge with a trail joining sharply from the left. Signs here indicate Middle Cove Loop to the left and Long Cove Loop to the right. Turn right and in a few hundred feet come to a fork and the start of the Long Cove Loop.

Bear right, skirt the shore of Long Cove Pond, and then follow a gently rolling course in a pine–oak forest. Close the very short loop, retrace your route to the next junction, and bear right on the Middle Cove Loop. After a path from the off-season parking area joins on the left, cross the off-season entrance road and follow a grassy path toward Middle Point Cove. Now meet a fork and the start of the Middle Cove Loop.

Angle left and traverse a dense oak woodland, soon approaching Middle Point Cove, a lovely, secluded body of water screened from view by a line of trees. The cove connects with Tisbury Great Pond via a narrow channel. Circle right and soon close the loop; then retrace your route to the four-way junction (mentioned at the start of paragraph four) near the staff residence and the former Scrubby Neck Schoolhouse.

Go straight through the four-way junction and continue about 100 feet to the next junction, where the road on the right also is closed to visitors. Bear left and soon reach

FLORA	FAUNA
Five distinct habitats characterize this refuge: sandplain grassland, heathland, scrub-oak shrubland, oak savanna, and oak forest. Close to the Atlantic shore, wind keeps the trees—mostly pitch pine and eastern red cedar—short. Farther inland, the black oaks, white oaks, and hickories attain respectable size. Low-growing, hardy shrubs dot the open terrain, including arrowwood, black huckleberry, bayberry, scrub oak, and dwarf sumac. Poison oak, Virginia creeper, wild grape, and berry vines thrive everywhere. The dunes are home to salt-spray rose, seaside goldenrod, beach pea, and dusty miller.	Check the skies for osprey, local nesters, and northern harriers on patrol, and for insect-catching swallows. Great blue herons, gulls, double-crested cormorants, and other waterbirds frequent the ocean and/or the ponds. Piping plovers, federally listed as threatened, nest just above the high-tide line on the outer beach.

a landing for kayaks and canoes. Most of the shore of Tisbury Great Pond is private, and this is one of the few places paddlers can land. To your right is a sandbar, sometimes filled with gulls and cormorants, guarding the entrance to Middle Point Cove.

Continue past the landing to the foot of a low dune, and then follow the trail, now a mowed swath, as it swings left. Soon rejoin the dirt road you were on earlier. If you are returning to the summer parking area, turn right and retrace your route by crossing the dune, turning left at the beach and then turning left again after about 0.5 mile.

If you are returning to the off-season parking area, turn left and walk about 0.3 miles to the four-way junction you were at earlier—the road going straight is closed to visitors. Two buildings are nearby. The larger is a staff residence, and the smaller is the Scrubby Neck Schoolhouse. Bear right on a grassy dirt road and soon meet a short trail that goes left to the off-season parking area.

DIRECTIONS

June 15–September 15: From the intersection of Edgartown–West Tisbury and Waldron Bottom roads in West Tisbury, take Waldron Bottom Road (paved, then dirt) southwest for 1.3 miles; then turn left on Scrubby Neck Road. Go 0.1 mile, turn right on Hughe's Thumb Road, and go another 1.2 miles to a gatehouse. A large dirt parking area is just ahead. The trailhead is on the southwest end of the parking area.

September 16–June 14: From the intersection of Edgartown–West Tisbury and Deep Bottom roads, take Deep Bottom Road southwest for 0.6 miles to a fork. Bear left, then left again at the next fork to get on Scrubby Neck Road. Go 0.3 miles to Thumb Point Road, turn right, and go another 1.3 miles (bearing left at all intersections) to the off-season parking area, left. The trailhead is on the southwest side of the parking area. *Note:* If you are using the off-season parking area, skip to the fifth paragraph of the description, above.

Shrubland Sally

GENERAL

DISTANCE 3.9 miles

TYPE OF WALK Loop

DIFFICULTY Moderate

TIME TO WALK 2–3 hours

MAPS *Manuel F. Correllus State Forest,* Massachusetts Department of Environmental Management; *Vineyard Haven,* USGS

SCENERY Forest, grassland, shrubland

EXPOSURE TO SUN Partial

TRAIL TRAFFIC Moderate

TRAIL SURFACE(S) Dirt, paved

TRAILS OPEN All year

FEES/PASSES None

FACILITIES None

TRAIL USE

BICYCLES Allowed; must yield to walkers and equestrians

DOGS Allowed on leash

HUNTING Allowed in season, generally from mid-October through February; wear blaze orange when appropriate

HEALTH STATS

NUMBER OF STEPS 8,775

ESTIMATED CALORIES BURNED 418

DIRECTIONS TO TRAILHEAD

From the intersection of State and Old County roads in West Tisbury, take Old County Road southwest 1.9 miles to a parking area on the left, opposite a school.

From the intersection of Edgartown–West Tisbury and Old County roads in West Tisbury, take Old County Road north; then northeast, for 1.5 miles to a parking area on the right, opposite a school.

The trailhead is on the northeast corner of the parking area, at fire lane B, gate 22.

Note: The entrance road to forest headquarters, where a map and other information are available, is on the east side of Barnes Road, 1.5 miles north from its intersection with Edgartown–West Tisbury Road.

Manuel F. Correllus State Forest is a 5,100-acre tract in the center of Martha's Vineyard.

WALK SUMMARY

The 5,100-acre state forest that lies at the center of Martha's Vineyard is a dynamic place. Native and nonnative plants and the creatures that depend on them for survival eke out a hardscrabble existence on poor soils, buffeted by blustering winds, always at the mercy of both natural and human-caused disturbances. Walking the dirt roads and trails described below gives visitors a chance to learn about and appreciate the processes at work in a sandplain ecosystem.

DESCRIPTION

From the trailhead, follow a paved path to the paved bicycle trail, carefully cross it, and then gain a dirt fire lane that heads northeast. After about 0.2 miles, turn right on a single-track trail that leads

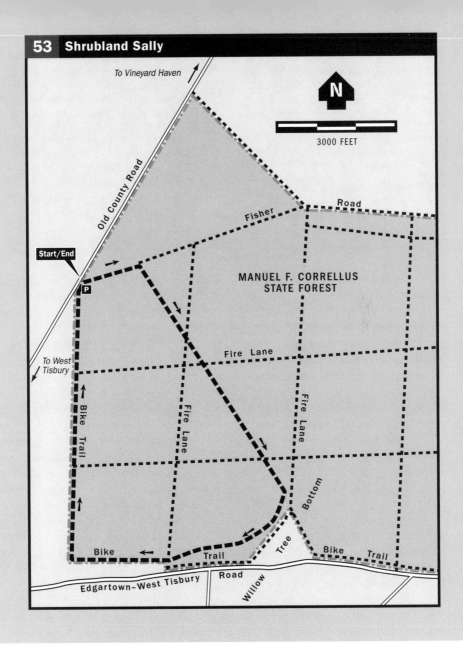

To Vineyard Haven

N

3000 FEET

Old County Road

Fisher   Road

Start/End

P

MANUEL F. CORRELLUS
STATE FOREST

To West
Tisbury

Fire   Lane

Bike   Trail

Fire   Lane

Fire   Lane

Bottom

Bike   Trail
Bike
Trail   Trail   Road

Tree

Willow

Edgartown–West Tisbury   Road

through a possibly unkempt corridor of trees and shrubs. Martha's Vineyard Airport is nearby, so don't be alarmed by low-flying planes.

Now the trail wanders through otherwise impenetrable thickets of low-growing shrubs, where there is no visible sign of human habitation. The solitude here, so close to busy roads and bicycle trails, is remarkable.

Created in 1908 as a reserve for the heath hen, a subspecies of the prairie chicken, which, unfortunately, was last seen in 1932, the forest soon saw extensive plantings of both white and red pines, thanks in part to Manuel F. Correllus, who was superintendent here from 1948 to 1987.

Because of disease, insect damage, and lack of thinning, neither species of tree produced marketable timber. Now these trees, which occupy about 500 acres, or roughly 10 percent of the state forest, represent a multifaceted problem—they prevent native species from thriving, create fuel for wildfires, and blow down in storms. The Department of Conservation and Recreation, which owns the forest, is considering logging, ironically, as one way to help restore the native sandplain ecosystem.

Cross a dirt road and continue on a single-track trail through a forest of pitch pine, a native species perfectly suited to this environment. The tall, rangy pines preside over a low-growing sea of shrubs, creating what is called a bilevel forest. After passing a meadow, cross the next dirt road and continue into a dense shrubland, where the trail is so narrow you almost need to put one foot directly in front of the other to proceed.

Another dirt road is ahead; after crossing it, reenter a forest and then descend gently through a clearing dotted with shrubs. Now climb through a wooded area, gently and then moderately, to gain a dirt road that joins from the left. Just beyond, at about the 1.5-mile point, you'll meet the paved bicycle trail. To avoid being run down, walk on a dirt trail that is, at first, just to the left of the bicycle trail, and then to its right.

Descend on a rolling course; then climb steeply right, away from the bicycle trail. Walk through forest on a curvy, undulating path that passes an unofficial trail, on your left, and soon meets the bike trail. Gain the paved trail by going straight, passing a dirt road on your right. After a few hundred feet the trail bends left and climbs moderately. (As a courtesy to bicyclists, please stay to the right while on the bicycle trail.)

Soon pass a trail on the left called Drifters Way, which leads to a youth hostel; a dirt road, also left, to a fire station; and a path on the lift signed WEST TISBURY. Continue straight through all these junctions. Now the bicycle trail turns right, passes a dirt road on the right, and then traverses terrain that is generally open on the left and wooded on the right. An unofficial trail cuts left, a dirt road goes right, and then the bicycle trail reaches the south side of the parking area, closing the loop.

Tisbury Great Pond

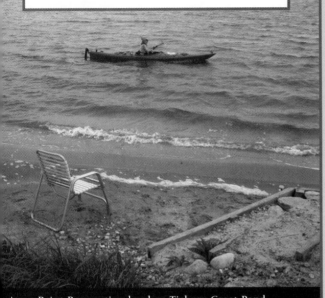

...piessa Point Reservation borders Tisbury Great Pond, ...popular boating spot.

WALK SUMMARY

This delightful walk explores a Land Bank reservation on the northeast side of Tisbury Great Pond, beside Tiah's Cove. Forested near the trailhead, the outer part of the route wanders through a restored meadow, formerly overgrown with shrubs and vines, that fringes the pond's shore. On the way back to the parking area, visitors stroll by a restored oak savanna, which may be alive with birdsong. Tisbury Great Pond is a popular boating area, and the parking areas here may fill early; please have an alternate destination in mind.

Note: Trail names (colors) on the latest Land Bank map may not correspond in all cases to signage or to names on older maps.

 KEY AT-A-GLANCE INFORMATION

GENERAL

DISTANCE 2.3 miles

TYPE OF WALK Balloon

DIFFICULTY Moderate

TIME TO WALK 1–2 hours

MAPS *Sepiessa Point Reservation,* Martha's Vineyard Land Bank Commission; *Tisbury Great Pond,* USGS

SCENERY Forest, meadow, pond

EXPOSURE TO SUN Partial

TRAIL TRAFFIC Moderate

TRAIL SURFACE(S) Dirt, sand

TRAILS OPEN All year

FEES/PASSES None

FACILITIES None

TRAIL USE

BICYCLES Allowed

DOGS Leashed May 1–August 31; leashed or under voice control September 1– April 30

HUNTING General hunting in season is allowed on this preserve, which is closed to the public during deer shotgun week, generally the first week in December; hunting is prohibited on Sunday and Monday, except during deer shotgun week, when hunting occurs on Monday.

HEALTH STATS

NUMBER OF STEPS 5,175

ESTIMATED CALORIES BURNED 246

DIRECTIONS TO TRAILHEAD

From the intersection of Edgartown–West Tisbury Road and New Lane in West Tisbury, take New Lane (which becomes Tiahs Cove Road) southeast 1.1 mile, past a sign on the left for Breezy Pines Farm. Turn right on dirt Clam Point Road and go 0.2 miles—passing an info board and a small parking area, both left—to a dirt parking area on the right (there is also a small parking area here on the left). The trailhead is on the northwest side of the parking area, signed CANOE DROP-OFF 100 FEET.

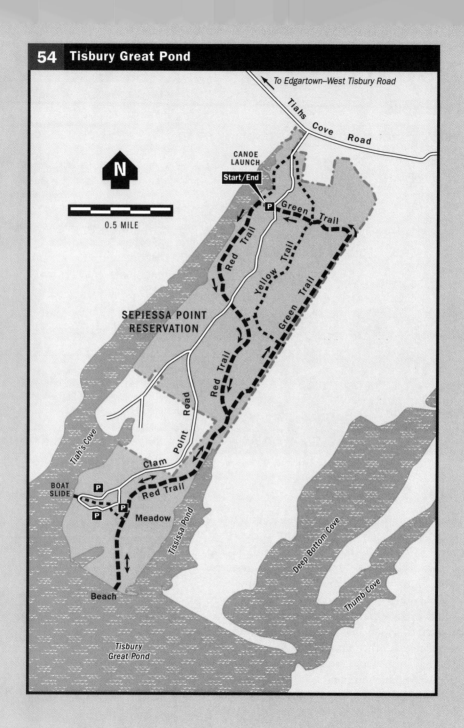

To Edgartown–West Tisbury Road

Tiahs Cove Road

CANOE
LAUNCH

Start/End

Green Trail

N

0.5 MILE

Red Trail

Yellow Trail

Green Trail

SEPIESSA POINT
RESERVATION

Red Trail

Clam Point Road

Tiah's Cove

BOAT
SLIDE

Red Trail

Meadow

Tississa Pond

Deep Bottom Cove

Thumb Cove

Beach

Tisbury
Great Pond

FLORA	FAUNA
Pitch pine, black oak, white oak, post oak, black cherry, and eastern red cedar are some of the common trees found here. The forest understory consists mostly of black huckleberry, highbush blueberry, lowbush blueberry, sweet pepperbush, swamp azalea, and sheep laurel. Arrowwood, bayberry, scrub oak, dwarf chestnut oak, poison ivy, and wild grape oak prefer more open areas. Wildflowers, including goldenrods, asters, wild indigo, and wood lily, decorate the grasslands in season.	Forest birds, often heard before they are seen, include eastern towhee, black-capped chickadee, and gray catbird. A red-tailed hawk or an osprey may be on patrol above the meadow at the southwest end of the reservation, and great black-backed gulls and double-crested cormorants often congregate near the shore of Tisbury Great Pond.

DESCRIPTION

From the trailhead, follow a single-track dirt trail gently downhill to a four-way junction. Ahead about 20 feet is Tiah's Cove (aka Tiah Cove), a narrow finger of water leading to Tisbury Great Pond. Turn left on the Red Trail, also called the Tiah's Cove Trail, which is marked with white squares nailed to trees. The trail bends left, passes a closed trail, right, and then reaches Clam Point Road (please use the trail system and not the road).

Cross the road and regain the trail, which now climbs gently and curves right. Soon meet a short connector, on the left, to the Yellow Trail, also called the Savanna Restoration Trail. Continue straight through a mostly oak forest with a low understory of shrubs. Bear right at a fork and almost immediately meet the Green Trail, which joins sharply from the left. Angle right to stay on the Red Trail.

Tississa Pond, which opens to Tisbury Great Pond, is to the left, behind trees. An osprey pole may be in use by a nesting pair of these fish-eating raptors. Glacially formed Tisbury Great Pond is isolated from the Atlantic Ocean by a barrier beach; storms and periodic dredging open a narrow channel in the beach, providing an influx of salt water.

Now join a dirt road, which angles in from the right, by going straight, and soon pass the Blue Trail, on the right. The grasslands here are the result of a successful land-management program to limit encroachment by shrubs and trees and thus restore and preserve hunting habitat for raptors such as hawks and owls. On a clear day, views across the beautiful open terrain stretch southward to the barrier beach fronting the ocean.

The Red Trail ends at a narrow strand of beach, which is private to the left and without much of a shoreline to the right. When ready, retrace your route to the junction of the Red and Green trails. Now walk straight on the Green Trail, marked with yellow squares nailed to trees, beside the reservation boundary, which is to the right.

Where the Yellow Trail, or Savanna Restoration Trail, goes left, continue straight. Notice how the woodland to the left, actively managed as a savanna, contrasts with the private land to the right. Open stands of trees interspersed with low understory shrubs create a habitat that attracts a wide variety of wildlife. In fact, scientists say that Native Americans used fire to help keep land open for hunting and to promote the growth of edible plants and seeds.

Pass a dirt road, on the left, and then follow the Green Trail as it curves left, descends gently, and crosses the Yellow Trail at a four-way junction. Now continue straight to Clam Point Road, cross it, and immediately arrive at the parking area.

GENERAL

DISTANCE 1.1 mile

TYPE OF WALK Balloon

DIFFICULTY Easy

TIME TO WALK 1 hour or less

MAPS *Ripley's Field Preserve,* Martha's Vineyard Land Bank Commission; *Vineyard Haven,* USGS

SCENERY Forest, meadow

EXPOSURE TO SUN Partial

TRAIL TRAFFIC Light

TRAIL SURFACE(S) Dirt

TRAILS OPEN All year

FEES/PASSES None

FACILITIES None

TRAIL USE

BICYCLES Allowed

DOGS Allowed on leash

HUNTING Archery and primitive-weapon hunting for deer only are allowed in season on this preserve; archery season for deer is generally mid-October to the end of November; primitive-weapon season for deer is generally mid-December to the end of December.

HEALTH STATS

NUMBER OF STEPS 2,475

ESTIMATED CALORIES BURNED 118

DIRECTIONS TO TRAILHEAD

From the intersection of State and Lamberts Cove roads in Tisbury (not in West Tisbury, where they also intersect), take Lamberts Cove Road northwest for 0.7 miles; then turn left on John Hoft Road (dirt). Go 0.1 mile to a small dirt parking area, left. The trailhead is on the south side of the parking area.

Forest and Field Foray

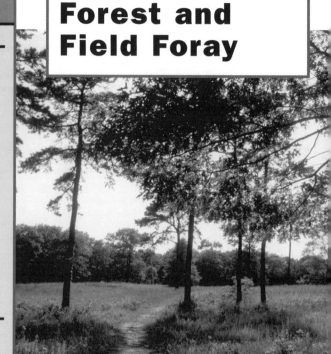

Ripley's Field Preserve features densely wooded forest and a large, open meadow.

WALK SUMMARY

This easy, well-shaded walk wanders through Ripley's Field, a lovely meadow graced by an old windmill and wildflowers in season, and then follows the 56-acre preserve's perimeter through a forest of mostly pine and oak.

DESCRIPTION

A sketch map at the trailhead shows the two trails, Red and Green, that traverse this 56-acre preserve. After studying the map, walk south on the Red Trail, a wide dirt path, into a pine–oak forest. Go several hundred feet to a junction with the Green Trail, which angles left. Continue straight and climb a short, rocky rise. Now follow a gently rolling course to the next junction, where the Red Trail begins a loop.

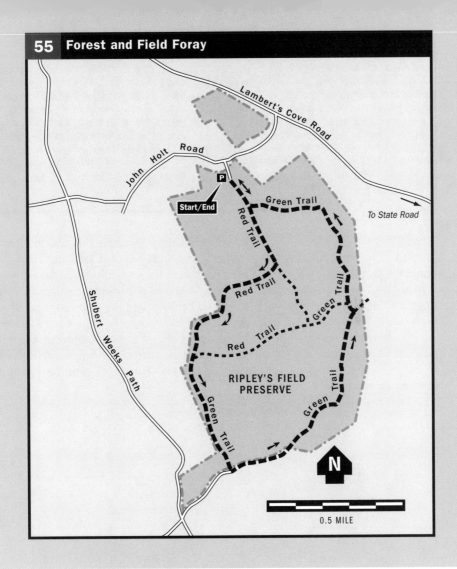

Turn right and emerge from forest into Ripley's Field, a meadow dotted with low shrubs and wildflowers. A lone, picturesque pine and a photogenic old windmill complete the scene. Returning to the woods, descend gently, then moderately, to a junction with the Green Trail. (To shorten the route, turn left here to stay on the Red Trail, and follow it back to the parking area.)

Walk straight, now on the Green Trail, and pass an unofficial trail, on the right, that exits the Land Bank property. This is a densely wooded, multilevel forest, with understories of various heights. By contrast, some of the Cape and Island's pine forests are bilevel, with the pines rarely reaching more than

50 feet, and the understory, usually black huckleberry, growing to only about 3 feet.

At a four-way junction—the unofficial trail going straight exits the Land Bank property—turn left to stay on the Green Trail, here a narrow dirt road, shown on the map as "Road to Chappaquonsett." The rocky road rises gently amid massive pitch pines to gain a ridgetop. The elevation is soon lost, however, and the road drops gently to a junction.

Follow the Green Trail by turning left; then almost immediately reach a four-way junction (the trail going right is unofficial). Continue straight and follow a roller-coaster course about 0.2 miles to a T-junction with the Red Trail. From here, turn right and retrace your route to the parking area.

Esker Escapade

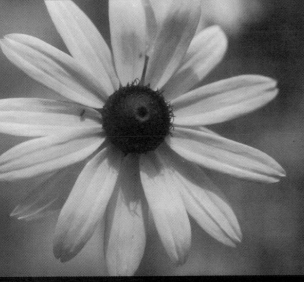

Wildflowers such as this black-eyed Susan are often found in open, grassy places.

KEY AT-A-GLANCE INFORMATION

GENERAL

DISTANCE 1.5 miles

TYPE OF WALK Balloon

DIFFICULTY Easy

TIME TO WALK 1 hour or less

MAPS *Tisbury Meadow Preserve,* Martha's Vineyard Land Bank Commission; *Vineyard Haven,* USGS

SCENERY Forest, meadow

EXPOSURE TO SUN Partial

TRAIL TRAFFIC Light

TRAIL SURFACE(S) Dirt

TRAILS OPEN All year

FEES/PASSES None

FACILITIES None

TRAIL USE

BICYCLES Allowed

DOGS Allowed on leash

HUNTING Archery and primitive-weapon hunting for deer only are allowed in season on this preserve. Archery season for deer is generally mid-October to the end of November. Primitive-weapon season for deer is generally mid-December to the end of December.

HEALTH STATS

NUMBER OF STEPS 3,375

ESTIMATED CALORIES BURNED 161

DIRECTIONS TO TRAILHEAD

From the intersection of State and Old County roads in West Tisbury, take State Road northeast for 1.2 miles; then turn right on the preserve's dirt entrance road. Go about 200 feet to a small dirt parking area. The trailhead is on the southeast side of the parking area.

From the intersection of State and Lamberts Cove roads in Tisbury, take State Road southwest 0.1 mile; then turn left on the preserve's dirt entrance road and follow the directions above.

WALK SUMMARY

This easy walk has something for everyone. Geology buffs will enjoy strolling atop an esker, which is a sand and/or gravel ridge formed by the movement of water associated with a melting glacier. Although there are a few pitch pines here, the forest consists mostly of hardwoods—oaks and other species—and this gives a richly wooded character to the terrain. *Note:* Trail names (colors) on the latest Land Bank map may not correspond in all cases to signage or to names on older maps.

DESCRIPTION

From the trailhead, walk past a bike rack and an information board, following the Yellow Trail, a dirt road that descends gently beside a restored 19th-century farmhouse, a pasture, and agricultural

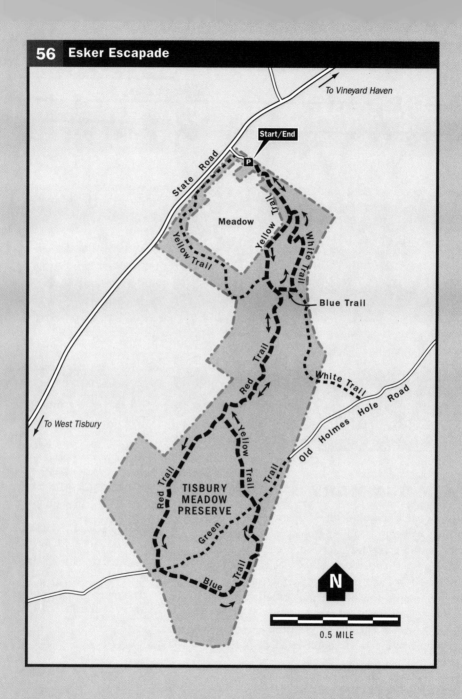

To Vineyard Haven

Start/End

State Road

Meadow

Yellow Trail

White Trail

Yellow Trail

Blue Trail

Red Trail

White Trail

To West Tisbury

Old Holmes Hole Road

Red Trail

Yellow Trail

Red Trail

TISBURY
MEADOW
PRESERVE

Green Trail

Blue Trail

N

0.5 MILE

fields, which are right. Stay on the Yellow Trail as it changes to a single-track trail and zigzags steeply uphill into a stand of pitch pines, black oaks, and eastern red cedars.

Emerge from the woods and follow a mowed path through a meadow to a junction where the White Trail departs left. Continue straight to the next junction, a fork. Angle left, walk about 50 feet, and then join the Red Trail by veering left. Now in a mixed-oak woodland, climb a set of dirt steps held in place by wood; then pass the Blue Trail, which goes left.

A moderate ascent leads to a ridgetop, where the trail follows a rolling course. Formed by meltwater percolating through a glacier and carrying debris with it, this ridge is called an esker. Now a moderate rocky descent leads past an unofficial trail, which goes right, to a junction with the Yellow Trail, on the left. Continue straight on the Red Trail; then curve left to meet dirt Old Holmes Hole Road at a four-way junction.

Cross the road and go straight, now on the Blue Trail. Soon an unofficial trail joins sharply on the right. Just ahead, the Blue Trail begins a gentle, curvy climb. Meet Old Holmes Hole Road again and cross it, now on the Yellow Trail. At a T-junction with the Red Trail, turn right and retrace your route to the junction with the Blue Trail, on the right. Turn right, go several hundred feet, and then turn left on the White Trail.

Traverse a hillside that drops left; then descend via S-bends toward the meadow. Make a short but moderate climb past an unofficial trail, which goes right. Rejoin the Yellow Trail, turn right, and retrace your route to the parking area.

KEY AT-A-GLANCE INFORMATION

GENERAL

DISTANCE 1.6 miles

TYPE OF WALK Balloon

DIFFICULTY Easy

TIME TO WALK 1 hour or less

MAPS *Vineyard Haven*, USGS

SCENERY Forest

EXPOSURE TO SUN Partial

TRAIL TRAFFIC Moderate

TRAIL SURFACE(S) Dirt

TRAILS OPEN All year

FEES/PASSES None

FACILITIES None

TRAIL USE

BICYCLES Trails not suitable for bicycles

DOGS Allowed on leash

HUNTING Not allowed

HEALTH STATS

NUMBER OF STEPS 3,600

ESTIMATED CALORIES BURNED 171

DIRECTIONS TO TRAILHEAD

From the intersection of State Road (Beach Street) and Main Street in Vineyard Haven, take Main Street north for 2 blocks (about 0.1 mile); then turn left on Center Street. Go 2 blocks (about 0.1 mile) to Franklin Street and turn right. Follow Franklin Street north for 1 mile to a dirt driveway on the right. Go several hundred feet to a very small dirt parking area, right. The trailhead is on the northeast corner of the parking area.

Woodsy Walk

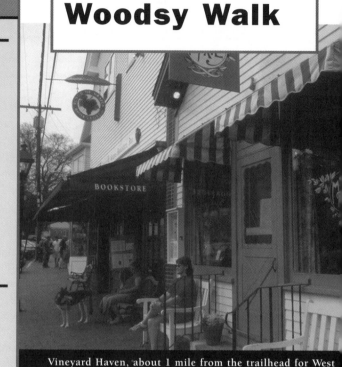

Vineyard Haven, about 1 mile from the trailhead for West Chop Woods, is a great place for shopping and a snack.

WALK SUMMARY

This 85-acre sanctuary, owned by the Sheriff's Meadow Foundation, provides a swath of wooded open space in an otherwise-developed, mostly residential area. Old Lighthouse Road, a dirt road, bisects the sanctuary and is designated the Red Trail, but note that there is also a single-track trail with the same name.

DESCRIPTION

This small sanctuary has four color-coded trails, which are shown on a rough sketch map at the trailhead. Follow the Blue Trail, which is the continuation of the dirt entrance road, southeast from the trailhead. Cross a power line right-of-way and enter a pine–oak forest on a wide, level dirt path.

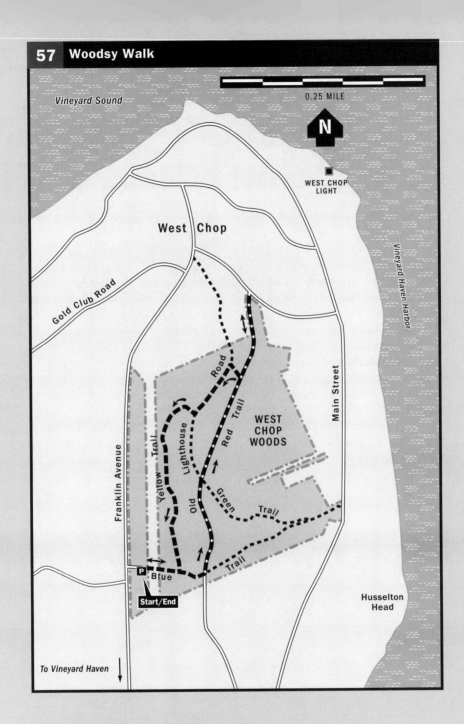

Vineyard Sound

0.25 MILE

N

WEST CHOP
LIGHT

West Chop

Vineyard Haven Harbor

Gold Club Road

Road

Red Trail

WEST
CHOP
WOODS

Main Street

Franklin Avenue

Yellow Trail

Lighthouse

Old

Green

Trail

Trail

P Blue

Start/End

Husselton
Head

To Vineyard Haven

Walk by the Yellow Trail, which goes left, and then pass a trail to a residential area on the right.

Now meet the Red Trail (Old Lighthouse Road) at a four-way junction. Turn left and follow a dirt road through a beautiful forest, where the tall pines and oaks are complemented by a low-growing understory. Go straight through the next junction, where the Green Trail joins from the right and a single-track trail, part of the Red Trail loop, angles left.

Continue straight on the dirt road and descend gently over rocky ground. Soon a gentle climb leads to a junction where the Red Trail loops in on the left. Walk straight and climb gently through an increasingly residential area to meet a dirt road at a T-junction. From here, retrace your route to the previous junction; then turn right on the Red Trail, a single-track trail. Bear sharply left at the next junction and then pass an unofficial trail heading right.

At a junction with the Yellow Trail, turn right and follow a gently rolling course that curves through forest to meet the Blue Trail. From here, turn right and retrace your route to the parking area.

Runway Ramble

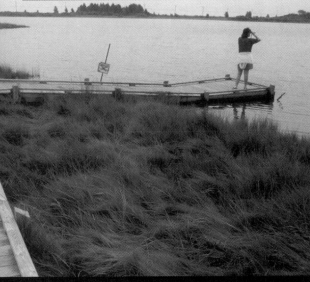

Farm Pond is the destination of this two-preserve walk, which starts at Trade Wind Fields Preserve.

WALK SUMMARY

An airport may seem an odd place to take a walk, but lack of development at Trade Wind Fields has preserved the sandplain grassland community, which is fast disappearing elsewhere on the Cape and Islands. A public trail links Trade Wind Fields with nearby Farm Pond Preserve, which has wetland habitats. Together the two preserves, which total nearly 100 acres, make a fine outdoor classroom for studying native plants. A universal-access trail, designed to accommodate wheelchairs, runs from the parking area to the trail system at the airport. Because the taxiway and runway are still in use, access by people and pets is prohibited. *Note:* Although the trails are signed with colored markers, the Land Bank map does not show the colors or the trail names.

 KEY AT-A-GLANCE INFORMATION

GENERAL

DISTANCE 3.1 miles

TYPE OF WALK Balloon

DIFFICULTY Moderate

TIME TO WALK 1–2 hours

MAPS *Trade Wind Fields Preserve, Farm Pond Preserve*, Martha's Vineyard Land Bank Commission; *Edgartown*, USGS

SCENERY Fields, forest, pond, shrub swamp

EXPOSURE TO SUN Partial

TRAIL TRAFFIC Moderate

TRAIL SURFACE(S) Dirt, sand

TRAILS OPEN All year

FEES/PASSES None

FACILITIES None

TRAIL USE

BICYCLES Allowed

DOGS Allowed on leash or under voice control

HUNTING Not allowed

HEALTH STATS

NUMBER OF STEPS 6,975

ESTIMATED CALORIES BURNED 332

DIRECTIONS TO TRAILHEAD

From the intersection of Edgartown-Vineyard Haven and County roads in Oak Bluffs, take County Road northeast for 1.7 miles; then turn right on a dirt road that leads to a large dirt parking area with handicapped parking. The trailhead is on the east side of the parking area, at its midpoint.

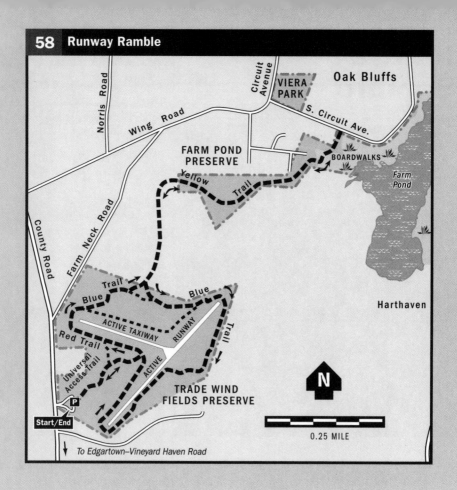

In the map:

Norris Road

Wing Road

Circuit Avenue

VIERA PARK

Oak Bluffs

S. Circuit Ave.

FARM POND PRESERVE

Yellow Trail

BOARDWALKS

Farm Pond

County Road

Farm Neck Road

Blue Trail

Blue Trail

ACTIVE TAXIWAY

ACTIVE RUNWAY

Red Trail

Universal Access Trail

Trail

Harthaven

N

TRADE WIND FIELDS PRESERVE

Start/End

P

0.25 MILE

To Edgartown–Vineyard Haven Road

DESCRIPTION

From the trailhead, walk northeast on a well-graded universal-access trail. Stay straight as trails join from the right, then left. Pass a rest bench and soon reach a T-junction with the Red Trail, which borders the active taxiway of Trade Wind Fields, a small airport. Turn left on the wide dirt path and pass the Green Trail, which is left. Eastern red cedars, a pioneering species, thrive in the airport's open fields.

At the northwest end of the taxiway, turn right, then right again to keep the taxiway on your right. Ignore a misplaced marker for the Blue Trail and keep a metal-roofed building on your left. At a junction just ahead, leave the Red Trail and veer left into a pitch-pine forest, now on the single-track Blue Trail. Reach a fork and angle left on the Yellow Trail, signed SCHOOL, FARM POND. Enjoy a level stroll cushioned by pine needles.

Pass a trail joining sharply from the right, which you will use later. Now your route swings left and parallels a dirt road. Yellow emblems on trees serve as trail markers but disappear when needed most—turn right to cross the dirt road, then right again, reversing direction. Oak Bluffs School, a sports field, and a paved road should be to the left.

Now follow the Yellow Trail, a wide dirt path, through a beautiful meadow to a junction. Here a short trail goes right to a boardwalk overlooking a shrub swamp. This makes a fine spot to study wetland plants, including water willow, a magenta-flowered shrub that "walks" its way into a pond or bog by means of arching branches with tips that form roots underwater.

Continue on the Yellow Trail, which penetrates a dense corridor of trees and shrubs. Traverse a wet area via a boardwalk; then reach a fork. Bear right and follow more boardwalk to the edge of marsh-fringed Farm Pond, where a rest bench awaits. The route soon turns left and reaches paved South Circuit Avenue. Now retrace your route on the Yellow Trail to Oak Bluffs School.

After making the U-turn to reverse direction (crossing the dirt road), veer left at the next junction. Soon merge with the Blue Trail as it joins sharply from the right. At the border of the active runway, join the wide path that skirts it, signed as the Blue Trail, by angling left. Now curve right, around the runway's northeast tip. Pass a fenced trail, left; then walk through an alley of pines and oaks beside a golf course, which is also left.

At the southwest end of the runway, make two right turns and walk northeast, keeping the runway on the right. At the junction with the universal-access trail, turn left and retrace your route to the parking area.

GENERAL

DISTANCE 1.4 miles

TYPE OF WALK Balloon

DIFFICULTY Easy

TIME TO WALK 1 hour or less

MAPS *Garrett Family Trail Guide*, Sheriff's Meadow Foundation; *Edgartown*, USGS

SCENERY Forest, marsh

EXPOSURE TO SUN None

TRAIL TRAFFIC Light

TRAIL SURFACE(S) Dirt, sand

TRAILS OPEN All year

FEES/PASSES None

FACILITIES None

TRAIL USE

BICYCLES Trail not suitable for bicycles

DOGS Allowed on leash

HUNTING Not allowed

HEALTH STATS

NUMBER OF STEPS 3,150

ESTIMATED CALORIES BURNED 150

DIRECTIONS TO TRAILHEAD

From the intersection of East Vineyard Haven and Beach roads in Edgartown, take East Vineyard Haven Road northwest for 0.6 miles to a roadside parking area, right. The trailhead is on the northeast side of the parking area.

Garrett Family Trail

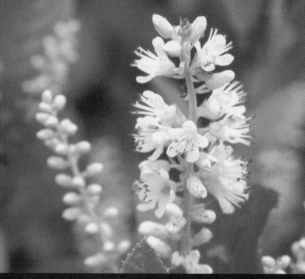

Sweet pepperbush is a common shrub whose spicy-sweet fragrance fills the woods in late summer.

WALK SUMMARY

This short, easy walk is the perfect answer to the question "Why preserve open space?" Located a few minutes from bustling Edgartown and sandwiched between busy highways and housing developments, the Caroline Tuthill Preserve offers a tranquil, relaxing place to enjoy nature. A self-guided trail leads visitors through pine–oak woods and alongside a salt marsh.

Boldface numbers in the description below refer to numbered markers along the trail, which are keyed to text in *Garrett Family Trail Guide*, a pamphlet that is usually available at the trailhead. A private road leading to private property crosses the trail at two places: please stay on the trail.

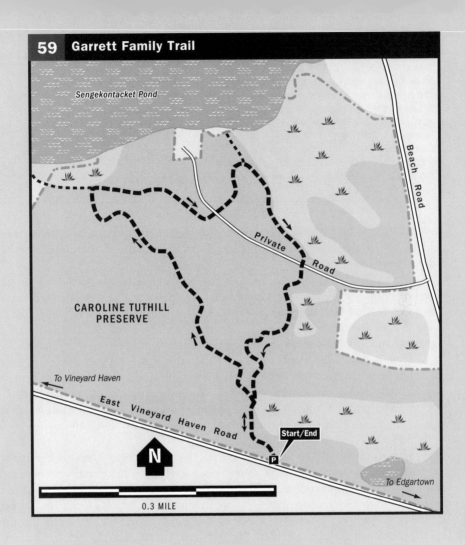

Sengekontacket Pond

Beach Road

Private Road

CAROLINE TUTHILL PRESERVE

To Vineyard Haven

East Vineyard Haven Road

N

Start/End

To Edgartown

0.3 MILE

DESCRIPTION

The self-guided nature trail here is named for Caroline Garrett Tuthill, who came to Martha's Vineyard in the early 1900s and, along with her sisters and other members of the Garrett family, worked to preserve the island's precious open spaces. This 150-acre preserve was a gift from John and Nora Tuthill to the Sheriff's Meadow Foundation, a local land trust.

From the trailhead, follow a sandy path into a wooded area. Climb gently; then descend to a junction, the start of a loop. Turn left, passing marker **1**, for lichens (left) and marker **2**, for fire adaptation in pitch pines (right). The open stands of pitch pine here are more typical of the Outer Cape than of

Martha's Vineyard, which is forested mostly in oak and other hardwoods. Tracing a level course, the trail meanders through the woods, passing marker **3,** which indicates pink lady's slipper orchids (left).

The route now curves right, crests a rise, and then descends gently to a junction, where an unofficial trail goes left. Continue straight past a trail post (white with a yellow band) and reach a four-way junction, in a clearing, with two unofficial trails. The trail going straight is a dead end. The trail going left meanders several hundred feet to a fork; the right-hand fork leads to a view of Sengekontacket Pond.

At the four-way junction mentioned above, turn right and pass marker **4,** for the transition from oak woods to wetland, left. Meet a dirt road (private), cross it, and then turn left and descend toward the pond. At a T-junction, an unofficial trail goes left. Turn right, walk to marker **5,** for salt marshes, and enjoy a limited view of the salt marsh that borders the pond. Now the trail curves right, recrosses the dirt road, and passes marker **6,** for two understory plants: spotted wintergreen and poison ivy.

After an unofficial trail joins from the left, your route zigzags moderately uphill to a modest summit, some 30 feet or so above sea level. Drop moderately over soft sand, and then follow a level course to close the loop at a junction. Just before closing the loop, you may notice a device that uses corn to attract deer, which are the primary hosts for the ticks that carry Lyme disease. When the deer try to eat the corn, they must first brush against material saturated with Permethrin, a tick repellent. Hopefully, this device and others like it will help control the spread of Lyme disease. From the junction, retrace your route to the parking area.

Jessica Hancock Trail

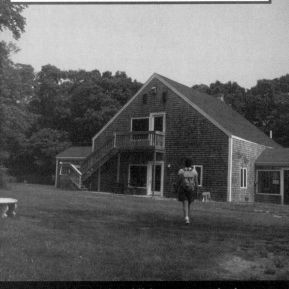

Visitors to Felix Neck Wildlife Sanctuary check in at The Barn, which has books, brochures, and displays.

 KEY AT-A-GLANCE INFORMATION

GENERAL

DISTANCE 1 mile

TYPE OF WALK Balloon

DIFFICULTY Easy

TIME TO WALK 1 hour or less

MAPS *Self-Guided Nature Walk to the Jessica Hancock Trail*, Massachusetts Audubon Society; *Edgartown*, USGS

SCENERY Forest, grassland, salt marsh, wetland

EXPOSURE TO SUN Partial

TRAIL TRAFFIC Moderate

TRAIL SURFACE(S) Dirt

TRAILS OPEN All year; sanctuary closes at 7 p.m.

FEES/PASSES Small fee for non-members of Massachusetts Audubon

FACILITIES Restrooms, nature center; water (seasonal)

TRAIL USE

BICYCLES Not allowed

DOGS Not allowed

HUNTING Not allowed

HEALTH STATS

NUMBER OF STEPS 2,250

ESTIMATED CALORIES BURNED 107

DIRECTIONS TO TRAILHEAD

From the intersection of East Vineyard Haven and Beach roads in Edgartown, take East Vineyard Haven Road northwest for 2.1 miles to Felix Neck Road, turn right, and go 0.7 miles to a large dirt parking area. The trailhead is on the north side of the parking area.

WALK SUMMARY

This lovely self-guided nature trail visits a variety of habitats, each with its own special array of native and nonnative plants. If you have time, consider also doing the "Woodland Wonderland" walk, described next in this book. Boldface numbers in the description below refer to numbered markers along the trail, which are keyed to text in a brochure available at the visitor center; some of the markers may be missing or hard to see. *Note:* Picnicking is permitted only in the parking area.

DESCRIPTION

From the trailhead, walk past an information board to the visitor center, housed in a building called The Barn. Check in here, pay a small entrance fee (for nonmembers), and spend a few minutes browsing

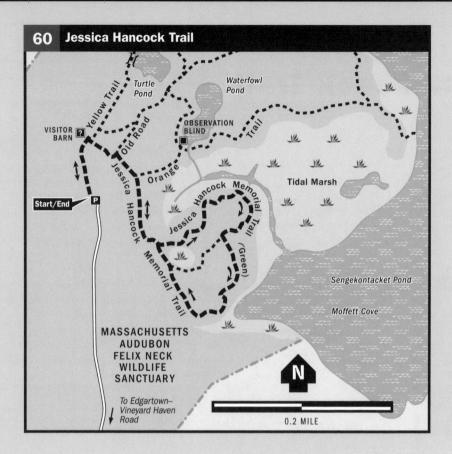

60 Jessica Hancock Trail

the books, brochures, and displays and perhaps chatting with a staff member or volunteer from the Massachusetts Audubon Society. When ready, step outside to find the start of three of the sanctuary's trails. While facing the door to the visitor center, you have the Yellow Trail going straight (northeast), skirting the right side of the barn. The Orange and Green trails, here joined, go right (southeast).

Choose the Orange/Green Trail and walk a few hundred feet across a lawn to Old Road, a dirt road. Marker **1**, nearby, is for the area's geologic history. Cross the road, passing marker **2** (change in the environment), and go another 100 feet or so to a fork, where the Orange and Green trails split. Bear right on a wide dirt path and come to markers **3** (an edge community where different habitats meet) and **4** (a row of trees called a "fence row").

Swing left at a fork and walk to marker **5**, which indicates an old pond and bog, fringed with cattails and other marsh vegetation. Entering a pine forest, the trail passes marker **6** (succession community), and then curves sharply left. Beyond marker **7** (intermediate and ground-cover communities), the trail narrows and wanders through a wooded area.

FLORA

Pitch pine, black oak, white oak, black cherry, tupelo, sassafras, eastern red cedar, and red maple are some of the trees found here. Shrubs include arrowwood, bayberry, black huckleberry, highbush blueberry, beach plum, winterberry, checkerberry, pasture rose, swamp azalea, sheep laurel, and sweet pepperbush. In the salt marsh grow salt hay, sea lavender, glasswort, marsh elder, and groundsel tree. A rich assortment of ferns and wetland plants thrive in moist areas near the old pond and bog. Poison ivy, Virginia creeper, grape, greenbrier, and bittersweet twine beside the trail.

FAUNA

Black-capped chickadee, red-winged blackbird, and northern flicker may noisily announce their presence. Gulls, terns, double-crested cormorants, and waterfowl frequent nearby Sengekontacket Pond. Check the skies for raptors, including osprey, on patrol.

Marker **8** (a wooded swamp) and marker **9** (the salt-marsh edge) are both on the left. At marker **10** (salt marsh), a short path leads left to the edge of a salt marsh bordering Sengekontacket Pond. After viewing the marsh, return to the main trail and turn left, continuing the clockwise loop. Pass marker **11,** which indicates the transition between woodland and wetland, and arrive at marker **12** (a mixed-oak community).

Now at a fork, angle left and walk about 100 feet to marker **13,** which indicates lichens in an old pasture community. There is a fine view of Sengekontacket Pond from here. Pass markers **14** (a cattail marsh) and **15** (a meadow community) before meeting a trail from the previous fork, which joins sharply from the right. Bear left and pass the old pond, marker **16,** which is fringed with ferns. Close the loop at a junction just ahead, continue straight, and retrace your route to the parking area.

KEY AT-A-GLANCE INFORMATION

GENERAL

DISTANCE 1 mile

TYPE OF WALK Balloon

DIFFICULTY Easy

TIME TO WALK 1 hour or less

MAPS *Felix Neck Wildlife Sanctuary,* Massachusetts Audubon Society; *Edgartown,* USGS

SCENERY Forest, marsh, pond

EXPOSURE TO SUN Partial

TRAIL TRAFFIC Moderate

TRAIL SURFACE(S) Dirt

TRAILS OPEN All year; sanctuary closes at 7 p.m.

FEES/PASSES Small fee for non-members of Massachusetts Audubon

FACILITIES Restrooms, nature center; water (seasonal)

TRAIL USE

BICYCLES Not allowed

DOGS Not allowed

HUNTING Not allowed

HEALTH STATS

NUMBER OF STEPS 2,250

ESTIMATED CALORIES BURNED 107

DIRECTIONS TO TRAILHEAD

From the intersection of East Vineyard Haven and Beach roads in Edgartown, take East Vineyard Haven Road northwest for 2.1 miles to Felix Neck Road, turn right, and go 0.7 miles to a large dirt parking area. The trailhead is on the north side of the parking area.

Woodland Wonderland

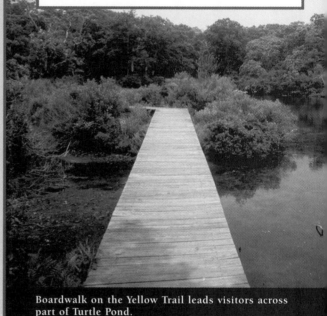

Boardwalk on the Yellow Trail leads visitors across part of Turtle Pond.

WALK SUMMARY

Massachusetts Audubon sanctuaries are great places to visit, and Felix Neck, located on a thumb of land poking north into Sengekontacket Pond, is no exception. The well-maintained trails, all wheelchair accessible, lead to a variety of habitats, including forest, meadow, salt marsh, and freshwater ponds, providing visitors with ample opportunities for nature study as well as exercise. Also at the sanctuary is the Jessica Hancock Trail, a self-guided nature walk with an accompanying brochure, which is described previously. *Note:* Picnicking is permitted only in the parking area.

DESCRIPTION

From the trailhead, walk past an information board to the visitor center, housed in a building called

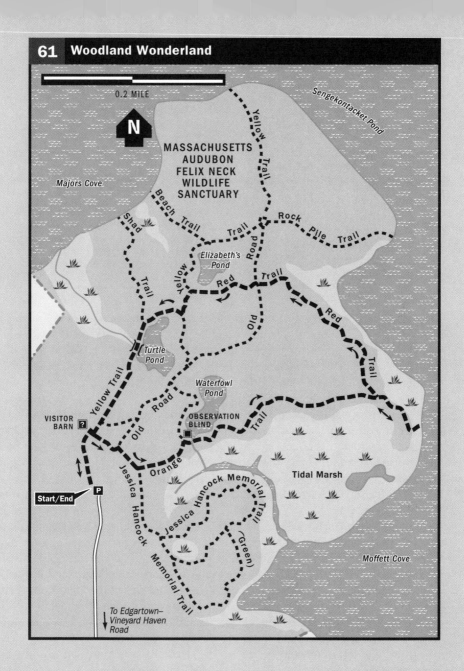

0.2 MILE

N

MASSACHUSETTS
AUDUBON
FELIX NECK
WILDLIFE
SANCTUARY

Majors Cove

Sengekontacket Pond

Shad Trail

Beach Trail

Yellow Trail

Rock Pile Trail

Elizabeth's Pond

Yellow Trail

Red Trail

Old Road

Red Trail

Turtle Pond

Waterfowl Pond

OBSERVATION BLIND

Old Road

VISITOR BARN

Yellow Trail

Orange

Jessica Hancock Memorial Trail

Tidal Marsh

Start/End

Jessica Hancock Memorial Trail

(Green)

Moffett Cove

To Edgartown–Vineyard Haven Road

The Barn. Check in here, pay a small entrance fee (for nonmembers), and spend a few minutes browsing the books, brochures, and displays and perhaps chatting with a helpful staff member or volunteer. When ready, step outside to find the start of three of the sanctuary's trails. While facing the door to the visitor center, you'll have the Yellow Trail going straight (northeast), skirting the right side of the barn. The Orange and Green trails, here joined, go right (southeast).

Choose the Orange/Green Trail and walk a few hundred feet across a lawn to Old Road, a dirt road. Cross the road and go another 100 feet or so to a fork, where the Orange and Green trails split. Bear left onto the Orange Trail and soon reach a junction beside human-made Waterfowl Pond, where there is an observation blind for bird-watching and photography. Turn right, cross the pond's outlet creek on a wooden bridge, and then enter a pine–oak forest. Views extend right to a salt marsh and ahead to Sengekontacket Pond.

At the next junction, where the Red Trail goes sharply left, stay on the Orange Trail by walking straight. Soon reach the shore of a wooded point, fringed with salt marsh, that arcs southeast into the pond. Sarsons Island, which supports colonies of great black-backed gulls, double-crested cormorants, and nesting American oystercatchers, is visible from here. When ready, retrace your route to the junction of the Orange and Red trails.

Now go straight on the Red Trail, skirting the pond shore. The trail climbs slightly, providing an overview of the pond, then curves left and descends to meet Old Road. Cross the road and follow a gently rolling course through an oak-dominated forest to a T-junction with the Yellow Trail. Turn left, go about 100 yards beneath stately oaks to a fork, and veer left to stay on the Yellow Trail. Turtle Pond is to the left, and the Shad Trail joins from the right.

Cross the outlet of Turtle Pond on a boardwalk; then emerge from forest into a meadow filled with butterfly weed, which sports orange flowers in summer. Turn right at a junction and walk a short distance to The Barn. From here, retrace your route to the parking area.

Spruce Circuit

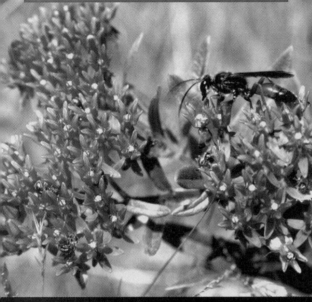
Although called butterfly weed, this species attracts many other insects, including wasps.

WALK SUMMARY

The "trails" in this 5,100-acre state forest consist of multiuse fire lanes, dirt paths, and paved bicycle trails. A magical world of pines, oaks, and non-native evergreens awaits the walker willing to leave the often busy bicycle trails and fire lanes and venture onto the sometimes overgrown dirt paths. This state forest also contains sandplain grasslands, a rapidly vanishing habitat that is home to a variety of rare plants and animals.

DESCRIPTION

From the trailhead, walk north on a dirt fire lane for about 15 feet to a paved bicycle trail. Turn left and walk along the right side of the trail, being alert for riders. The level trail runs through a shady corridor of trees and shrubs, parallel to the busy

KEY AT-A-GLANCE INFORMATION

GENERAL

DISTANCE 4.5 miles

TYPE OF WALK Loop

DIFFICULTY Moderate

TIME TO WALK 2–3 hours

MAPS *Manuel F. Correllus State Forest,* Massachusetts Department of Environmental Management; *Edgartown,* USGS

SCENERY Forest, grassland, shrubland

EXPOSURE TO SUN Partial

TRAIL TRAFFIC Moderate

TRAIL SURFACE(S) Dirt, paved, sand

TRAILS OPEN All year

FEES/PASSES None

FACILITIES None

TRAIL USE

BICYCLES Allowed; must yield to walkers and equestrians

DOGS Allowed on leash

HUNTING Allowed in season, generally from mid-October through February; wear blaze orange when appropriate

HEALTH STATS

NUMBER OF STEPS 10,125

ESTIMATED CALORIES BURNED 482

DIRECTIONS TO TRAILHEAD

From the intersection of Edgartown–West Tisbury and Barnes roads in Edgartown, take Edgartown–West Tisbury Road east for 1.6 miles to a parking area, left. Please don't block the fire gate with your car. The trailhead is on the north side of the parking area, at gate 2.

Note: The entrance road to forest headquarters, where a map and other information are available, is on the east side of Barnes Road, 1.5 miles north from its intersection with Edgartown–West Tisbury Road.

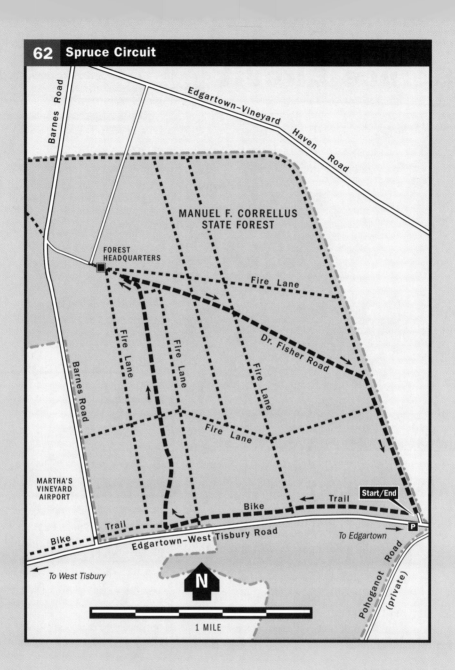

MANUEL F. CORRELLUS
STATE FOREST

FOREST
HEADQUARTERS

Fire Lane

Dr. Fisher Road

Fire Lane

Fire Lane

Fire Lane

Fire Lane

Fire Lane

Barnes Road

Barnes Road

Edgartown–Vineyard Haven Road

MARTHA'S
VINEYARD
AIRPORT

Bike

Trail

Bike

Trail

Start/End

P

Edgartown–West Tisbury Road

To Edgartown

Pohoganot Road
(private)

To West Tisbury

N

1 MILE

FLORA	FAUNA
Trees here include pitch pine, white pine, black oak, white oak, post oak, black cherry, bigtooth aspen, shadbush, gray birch, autumn olive, white spruce, and Norway spruce. Open, sandy areas favor shrubs such as scrub oak, dwarf chestnut oak, dwarf sumac, arrowwood, black huckleberry, bayberry, bearberry, low-bush blueberry, and chokeberry. Just off the trail (and sometimes on it) grow vines—poison ivy, greenbrier, berries—and ferns. Some wildflowers at home here are fleabane, dogbane, chicory, wild indigo, bush clover, yarrow, butterfly weed, and goldenrod.	Ospreys, red-tailed hawks, and American crows may be circling overhead, while the forest and underbrush may hold black-capped chickadees, eastern towhees, nuthatches, and sparrows.

Edgartown–West Tisbury Road. Walk past gate 3 and then a trail, both right. Just beyond gate 4, which is left, the trail makes a swooping descent into a slight valley.

Where the trail straightens and before it starts to climb, turn right onto an unsigned and possibly overgrown dirt trail. Now enter a secluded, densely forested realm, where stands of white spruce, unusual on the Cape and Islands, border the trail, along with low-growing oaks and black huckleberry. Go straight through a four-way junction, enjoying a level walk on a hard-packed dirt trail.

Soon pass a large clearing to your right, mostly screened by trees. Cross a fire lane and continue on the trail, directly beneath the flight path of small planes approaching the island's airport. At about 2 miles, emerge from forest into a sea of scrub oak and dwarf chestnut oak. At a four-way junction, go straight, now on a dirt road that skirts an open area of grassland, which is right. Curve left and meet another dirt road joining sharply from the right.

As the road bends left, turn right on a trail cutting through a line of trees and shrubs. This trail is called Dr. Fisher Road on the park map; according to a park ranger, it is one of the oldest walking paths on the island. (If you come to a sandpit on the left, you've gone too far and missed the trail; forest headquarters is about 0.25 miles ahead on the road.)

Along the way, unofficial trails diverge left and right: ignore these to stay on the described route. Cross a fire lane and traverse a beautiful forest of nonnative Norway and white spruce. Cross the next fire lane and stroll through groves of white pines. At the third fire lane, bear right and follow it over mostly open ground, past a dirt road signed D12, to the parking area.

GENERAL

DISTANCE 2 miles

TYPE OF WALK Out-and-back with a tiny loop

DIFFICULTY Moderate

TIME TO WALK 1 hour or less

MAPS *Poucha Pond Reservation,* Martha's Vineyard Land Bank Commission; *Edgartown,* USGS

SCENERY Forest, pond, salt marsh

EXPOSURE TO SUN Partial

TRAIL TRAFFIC Light

TRAIL SURFACE(S) Dirt, gravel

TRAILS OPEN All year

FEES/PASSES None

FACILITIES None

TRAIL USE

BICYCLES Allowed

DOGS Allowed on leash or under voice control

HUNTING General hunting in season is allowed on this preserve, which is closed to the public during deer shotgun week, generally the first weekend in December; hunting is prohibited on Sunday and Monday, except during deer shotgun week, when hunting occurs on Monday.

HEALTH STATS

NUMBER OF STEPS 4,500

ESTIMATED CALORIES BURNED 214

DIRECTIONS TO TRAILHEAD

From the Edgartown–Chappaquiddick ferry, take Chappaquiddick Road southeast 2.5 miles. Where Dike Road goes straight, turn right to stay on Chappaquiddick (School) Road. Go 0.8 miles; then turn left on Pocha (Wasque) Road. Go 0.9 miles and turn left onto a dirt road that leads about 100 feet to a small dirt parking area, which has handicapped parking. The trailhead is on the south corner of the parking area.

Salt Marsh Stroll

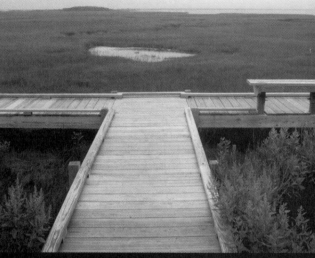

Platform just off the White Trail affords views of a large salt marsh bordering Poucha Pond.

WALK SUMMARY

This easy walk, best undertaken off-season, when the weather is cool and the biting insects gone, explores a 147-acre reservation perched on the shore of Poucha Pond. The pond is a body of saltwater connected to Cape Poge Bay by a narrow channel that flows under the infamous Chappaquiddick Island dike bridge. The reservation's trail system samples a variety of habitats, including forest, shrubland, and salt marsh.

DESCRIPTION

Passing an information board with a sketch map showing the reservation's color-coded trails, follow the White Trail for 100 feet or so to a rest bench, with fine views extending across shrubland, forest, and salt marsh to Poucha Pond. Beyond the pond is

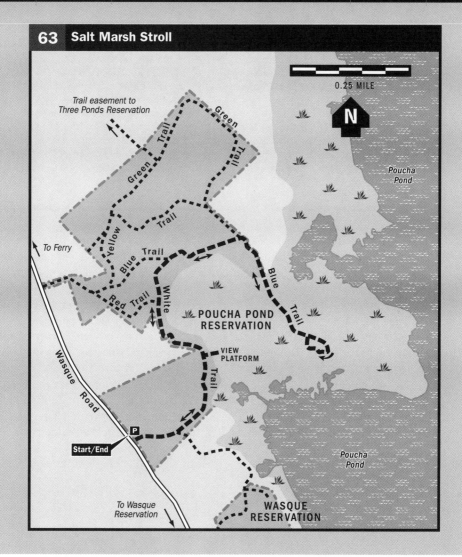

63 **Salt Marsh Stroll**

0.25 MILE

N

Trail easement to
Three Ponds Reservation

Green Trail

Green Trail

Poucha
Pond

Trail

Yellow Trail

To Ferry

Blue Trail

Blue Trail

Red Trail

White Trail

**POUCHA POND
RESERVATION**

VIEW
PLATFORM

Trail

Wasque Road

P

Start/End

Poucha
Pond

To Wasque
Reservation

**WASQUE
RESERVATION**

a barrier beach that fronts on Muskeget Channel, the waterway separating Martha's Vineyard and Nantucket. (From the trailhead to the rest bench, the White Trail is a universal-access trail.)

Now descend gently on a dirt trail through an area of scrub vegetation, soon meeting a trail, right, to Wasque Reservation. A walk in this reservation, which is on the southeast corner of Chappaquiddick Island, is described elsewhere in this book (Ocean's Edge, page 242). Curve left, still descending, and soon enter forest. At a junction just ahead, a short trail goes right to a viewing platform overlooking a salt marsh.

The White Trail continues through a junglelike area, where a riot of vegetation lurks just off the trail and boardwalks cover patches of possibly wet ground. The now-level route passes an unofficial trail on your left, turns right, and soon reaches a junction. Here the White Trail ends and the Red Trail goes left and straight. Continue straight to the next junction and merge with the Blue Trail by going straight, then bending right.

At a T-junction where the Yellow Trail goes left, turn right to stay on the Blue Trail. Immediately join a dirt road by angling right; to the left the road is gated and signed PRIVATE PROPERTY. Ahead, another road, also marked as private, goes left. Now your road, which may flood at high tide, crosses an expanse of salt marsh, with shallow pools of water, called salt pannes, on both sides.

The road briefly crosses a small, densely wooded island, then traverses another lobe of salt marsh. At the next island, also wooded, the return leg of the Blue Trail's terminal loop joins on the right. Go straight to the next junction and bear right. Close the short loop; then retrace your route on the Blue, Red, and White trails to the parking area.

Brines Pond Preserve

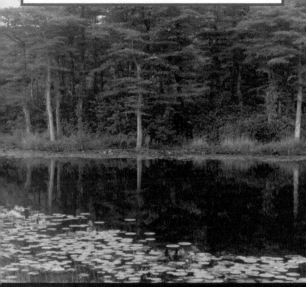

Brines Pond is a part of Three Ponds Reservation, administered by the Martha's Vineyard Land Bank Commission.

GENERAL

DISTANCE 1 mile

TYPE OF WALK Balloon

DIFFICULTY Easy

TIME TO WALK 1 hour or less

MAPS *Three Ponds Reservation*, Martha's Vineyard Land Bank Commission; *Edgartown*, USGS

SCENERY Forest, pond

EXPOSURE TO SUN Partial

TRAIL TRAFFIC Light

TRAIL SURFACE(S) Dirt

TRAILS OPEN All year

FEES/PASSES None

FACILITIES None

TRAIL USE

BICYCLES Allowed

DOGS Allowed on leash or under voice control

HUNTING General hunting in season, except for waterfowl, is allowed on this preserve, which is closed to the public during deer shotgun week, generally the first weekend in December; hunting is prohibited on Sunday and Monday, except during deer shotgun week, when hunting does occur on Monday.

HEALTH STATS

NUMBER OF STEPS 2,250

ESTIMATED CALORIES BURNED 107

DIRECTIONS TO TRAILHEAD

From the Edgartown–Chappaquiddick ferry, take Chappaquiddick Road southeast for 1.6 miles; then turn right at the Chappaquiddick Community Center entrance, a dirt road. Stay right at the start of a loop; then go straight where the loop curves sharply left. Go about 100 feet or so to a parking area on your right; if this is full, there is another parking area just ahead. The trailhead is on the southeast corner of the first parking area.

WALK SUMMARY

Enjoy this short, woodsy stroll in the fall, when the tupelo trees on the island in Brines Pond take on their autumn hues. The trail network here connects with trails leading to other nearby preserves, making longer rambles possible.

Note: Trail names (colors) on the latest Land Bank map may not correspond in all cases to signage or to names on older maps.

DESCRIPTION

From the trailhead, walk gently downhill on a dirt road to the second parking area, which is bordered by a split-rail fence. Bear left into an open field, where there is an information board. Facing the board, you have Brines Pond on your left and the Yellow Trail (signed with a red trail marker on a pine

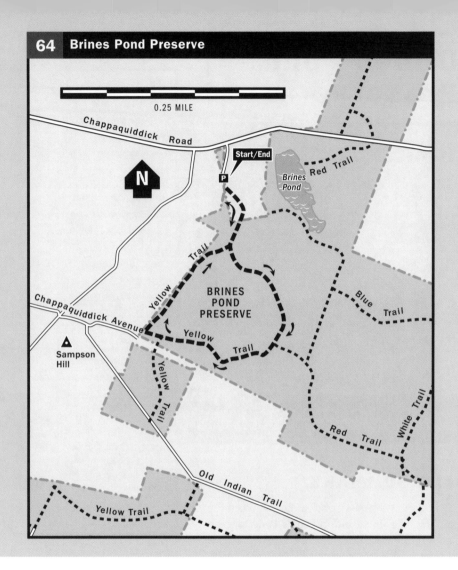

0.25 MILE

Chappaquiddick Road

N

Start/End

P

Red Trail

Brines Pond

Trail

Yellow

BRINES POND PRESERVE

Yellow Trail

Blue Trail

Chappaquiddick Avenue

Yellow Trail

Sampson Hill

Red Trail

White Trail

Old Indian Trail

Yellow Trail

tree) just ahead and slightly right. A small island at the pond's north corner is home to a stand of tupelo trees, whose leaves make a colorful show in fall.

Follow the Yellow Trail, a dirt road, into a pine–oak forest. After about 100 yards, turn left where the Yellow Trail splits to begin a loop. Enjoy a gently rolling stroll to the next junction, and pass the Green Trail (not on the map), which departs right. Continue straight to a T-junction (not on the map) and turn right onto a wide path.

Angle right at an upcoming fork and climb gently to meet the Green Trail at another T-junction. Turn left to stay on the Yellow Trail; then begin a clockwise circuit of a large, open field, mostly screened from view by trees. Roll gently along to meet the Red Trail, which joins sharply from the left. Just ahead is a fork; stay right and remain true to the Yellow Trail, which skirts the field. Close the loop at a junction and then retrace your route to the parking area.

Ocean's Edge

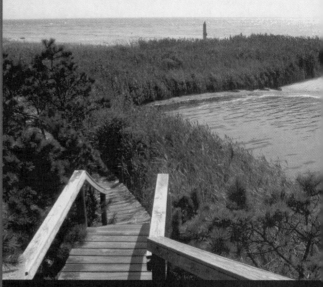

Steps and boardwalk lead past the east end of Swan Pond to Wasque Point.

WALK SUMMARY

This easy walk explores a compact but surprisingly varied reservation on the southeast corner of Chappaquiddick Island. Habitats here include pine–oak forest, heathland, and grassland. The mostly level route skirts a lovely pond, visits a sandy beach, and then wanders through wooded and open areas away from the water. This walk is best enjoyed off-season, when the weather is cool and biting insects not a problem.

DESCRIPTION

Two routes diverge from the trailhead, where several interpretive panels explain the island's geological past. To the right, a 500-foot boardwalk goes southwest to a low dune overlooking the Atlantic Ocean. To the left, a sandy road, signed TRAIL, skirts

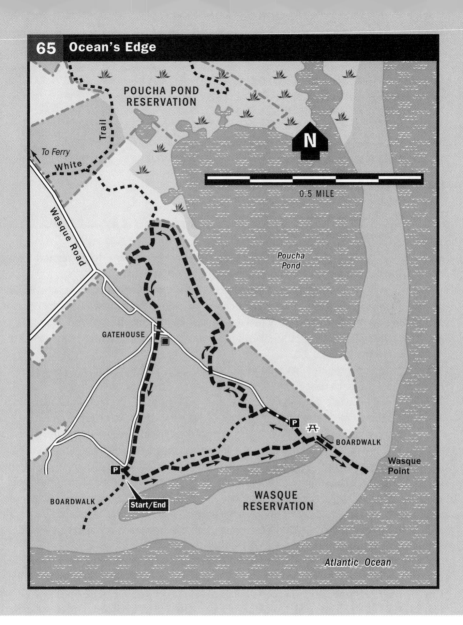

Swan Pond, which is home to gulls, double-crested cormorants, shorebirds, and a variety of waterfowl. Turn left and walk about 0.1 mile to a fork, enjoying open views across wind-pruned scrub vegetation.

Stay right, still on a dirt road, and pass a rest bench overlooking the long, narrow pond. Soon after the other branch of the fork rejoins on the left, wander through a corridor, then a tunnel, of trees and shrubs, with occasional "windows" on the right, each with its own rest bench. A picnic area and the

FLORA	FAUNA
Joining the wind- and salt-tolerant pitch pines are a few other hardy species of trees, including eastern red cedar, white oak, and black cherry. Shrubs such as scrub oak, bayberry, arrow-wood, salt-spray rose, and bearberry thrive in the dry, sandy soil, along with dune plants such as dusty miller and sea rocket. Poison ivy and Virginia creeper thread their way along the ground. Open grasslands feature asters, goldenrods, and other wildflowers, which provide food for migrating monarch butterflies.	Swan and Poucha ponds attract gulls, double-crested cormorants, wading birds, shorebirds, and waterfowl. Raptors such as osprey and northern harriers patrol the skies, along with insectivores such as eastern kingbirds and bluebirds. Various species of butterflies, including migrating monarchs, may be found in the sandplain grasslands and heathlands.

start of a boardwalk to the beach are at the Edmund Leland overlook, named for a former landowner whose descendants still own property nearby.

To reach the beach, follow a boardwalk and steps downhill past the northeast end of Swan Pond. The narrow, sandy strand near Wasque Point makes a perfect picnic or sunbathing spot, but dangerous currents caused by the meeting of the Atlantic Ocean and Muskeget Channel prohibit swimming here. When ready, retrace your route to the overlook and picnic area.

From the picnic area, go straight (northwest), away from the water, and gain a dirt road. Follow the road past the anglers parking area, which is to your right. After several hundred feet, veer left on a wood-chip trail. Walk another 200 feet or so to a junction and turn right. A short stretch of pine–oak forest soon gives way to open terrain.

This reservation features two types of nonforested uplands—coastal heathland and sandplain grassland. Grasslands and heathlands are mostly open, grassy areas dotted with low-growing shrubs and other plants. They differ primarily in the percentage of shrub-covered land, with heathlands having more shrubs than grasslands. Land managers use a variety of techniques, including prescribed burning, grazing, mowing, and brush-cutting, to prevent encroachment by trees and large shrubs. These habitats are rapidly disappearing on the Cape and Islands, and preserving them ensures the survival of many plants and animals, some of them rare.

At about the 1-mile point, cross the dirt road you were on a few minutes ago; then regain the trail, here a path of mowed grass. The large body of water ahead is Poucha Pond, which is connected by a narrow channel to Cape Poge Bay. The Martha's Vineyard Land Bank Commission owns land bordering part of Poucha Pond, and a walk there is described elsewhere in this book (see Salt Marsh Stroll, page 236).

Reentering forest, the trail follows a gently rolling course to a four-way junction. Continue straight and then bend sharply left at a split-rail fence. A rest bench in a clearing signals the start of a swerving-but-level stretch, which soon reaches the entrance gatehouse. From here, follow the dirt road you drove on earlier and walk about 0.4 miles south to the parking area, staying left at the fork signed PARKING AREA.

Nantucket

KEY AT-A-GLANCE INFORMATION

GENERAL

DISTANCE 2.4 miles

TYPE OF WALK Balloon

DIFFICULTY Moderate

TIME TO WALK 1–2 hours

MAPS *Middle Moors Properties Map*, Nantucket Conservation Foundation; *Siasconset*, USGS

SCENERY Heathland, shrubland

EXPOSURE TO SUN Full

TRAIL TRAFFIC Moderate

TRAIL SURFACE(S) Dirt, sand

TRAILS OPEN All year

FEES/PASSES None

FACILITIES None

TRAIL USE

BICYCLES Allowed only on well-established roads, not on single-track trails

DOGS Allowed on leash

HUNTING Allowed in season

HEALTH STATS

NUMBER OF STEPS 3,600

ESTIMATED CALORIES BURNED 171

DIRECTIONS TO TRAILHEAD

From the intersection of Milestone and Polpis roads (west of Nantucket Town), take Polpis Road northeast for 3 miles to Altar Rock Road, a dirt road directly opposite Quaise Road. Turn right, cross a paved bike trail, and go 0.1 mile, passing a small dirt parking area, on the left, to a second small dirt parking area, also left. (If this parking area is full, return to the first one.) The trailhead is on the east side of the parking area, where it meets Altar Rock Road.

Moorish Delight

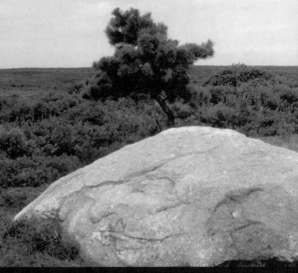

A rock and a lone tree are characteristic of the stark landscape around Altar Rock.

WALK SUMMARY

This moderate walk is but a brief introduction to the Middle Moors, a vast tract of rolling hills, kettle ponds, and cranberry bogs in the heart of Nantucket. Although John Muir derided sheep as "hoofed locusts" for their decimation of Yosemite's vegetation, sheep and other livestock grazing on Nantucket in the 1800s, along with poor soils and salty air, helped create the grasslands and heathlands enjoyed today by walkers, bicyclists, birders, nature enthusiasts, and others. Land managers use various techniques to help keep land free from encroaching trees and shrubs.

DESCRIPTION

From the trailhead, walk gently uphill on Altar Rock Road, passing after about 0.2 miles a road on

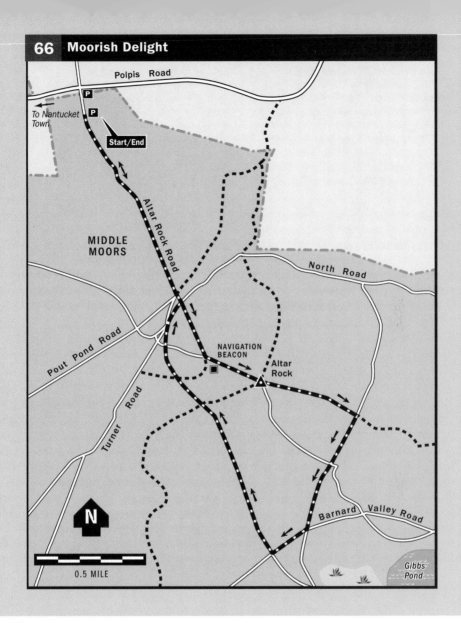

the right. A gentle descent leads to a fork, where the road divides into two parallel branches that remain within a few feet of each other. Continue straight over mostly level ground to a junction, where two dirt roads join on the left, and another two join on the right. Now follow Altar Rock Road as it rises on a gentle grade toward a communication facility. Near the facility is a junction where two dirt roads join from the right, one sharply, the other less so.

Continue uphill on Altar Rock Road, which makes a slight jog to the left and then straightens. Expansive views begin to reveal the extent of preserved open space on Nantucket, where more than 45 percent of the island's acreage is protected by private and public conservation interests. Middle Moors is a 4,000-acre collection of contiguous parcels located in the center of the island, most of which are owned by the Nantucket Conservation Foundation.

Pass a trail on your right, which leads uphill to a glacial boulder. The road soon tops out on Altar Rock, a 100-foot-high hill that is the island's fourth highest point. From this commanding vantage point, which offers 360-degree views, a beautiful vista extends northward across Nantucket Harbor to the lighthouse at Great Point. Just right of the crest is a small dirt parking area, from where a dirt road goes south and a very rough trail descends to the west. A metal plaque bolted to a nearby rock memorializes Henry Coffin (1807–1900), a lifelong island resident.

Continue on Altar Rock Road, keeping the parking area on your right, and follow a rolling course over eroded ground. In places, single-track trails diverge from the dirt road: ignore these to stay on the described route. A long descent leads past a dirt road, on the left, to a four-way junction. Turn right, go about 50 feet, and then continue straight through another four-way junction. Walk several hundred yards to a five-way junction and again continue straight (southwest).

A level stroll across open terrain leads to a sharply angled four-way junction. Bear right and climb on a gentle grade. Gibbs Pond, which provides water for nearby Milestone Cranberry Bog, is to the left. At the next junction, turn right and continue winning back a bit of elevation, in some places over soft sand. Pass a barricaded dirt road, on the right, and then meet a single-track trail at a four-way junction. Continue straight; the communication facility you passed earlier is about 100 yards to your right.

Stay straight where a dirt road veers right, and in about 60 feet come to a four-way junction. Again stay straight and walk several hundred yards to the next junction, also four-way. Proceed straight through this junction, almost immediately pass a road veering left, and in about 150 feet merge with a road joining sharply from the left. Curving right, the road forks, but both forks stay close together and lead several hundred feet to Altar Rock Road. Close the loop at the junction, turn left, and retrace your route on Altar Rock Road to the parking area.

Miacomet Pond

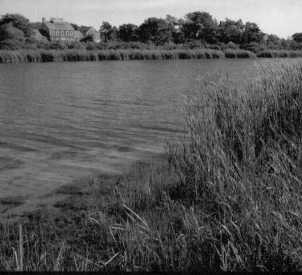

Burchell property borders Miacomet Pond, a narrow body of water southwest of Nantucket Town.

 KEY AT-A-GLANCE INFORMATION

GENERAL

DISTANCE 1.6 miles

TYPE OF WALK Balloon

DIFFICULTY Easy

TIME TO WALK 1 hour or less

MAPS *Siasconset*, USGS

SCENERY Forest, grassland, heathland, shrubland

EXPOSURE TO SUN Partial

TRAIL TRAFFIC Light

TRAIL SURFACE(S) Dirt, sand

TRAILS OPEN All year

FEES/PASSES None

FACILITIES None

TRAIL USE

BICYCLES Allowed

DOGS Allowed on leash

HUNTING Not allowed

HEALTH STATS

NUMBER OF STEPS 3,375

ESTIMATED CALORIES BURNED 161

DIRECTIONS TO TRAILHEAD

From the intersection of Surfside and Bartlett roads (south of Nantucket Town), take Bartlett Road southwest for 0.5 miles to Mizzenmast Road. Turn left and go 0.3 miles to a dirt parking area at the end of the road, on the right (there is also a smaller, paved parking area on the left). The trailhead is on the west side of the dirt parking area.

WALK SUMMARY

This short stroll visits a 42-acre property owned by the Nantucket Islands Land Bank, a land-acquisition program funded by a transfer fee on the sale of Nantucket real estate. This program, started in 1983 and said to be the first of its kind in the United States, has protected nearly 2,500 acres on Nantucket. The sandplain habitat here includes pine forest, grassland, heathland, and shrubland bordering Miacomet Pond.

DESCRIPTION

From the trailhead, enter a woodland of pines and shrubs on a sandy single-track trail that meanders over mostly level ground to a junction, where a path heads right. Open fields and a residential area are also right. Continue straight and gently uphill;

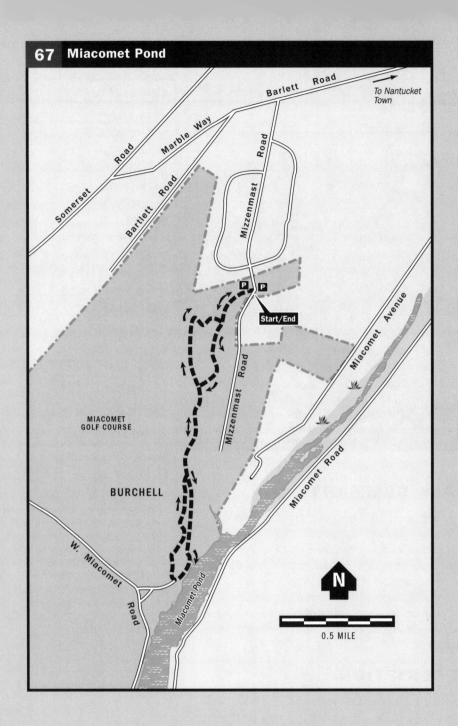

To Nantucket Town

Barlett Road

Somerset Road

Marble Way

Bartlett Road

Mizzenmast Road

P P

Start/End

Mizzenmast Road

Miacomet Avenue

MIACOMET GOLF COURSE

BURCHELL

W. Miacomet Road

Miacomet Pond

Miacomet Road

N

0.5 MILE

then walk on level ground past a rest bench on your right. Resume a gentle climb through a beautiful pine forest to where a trail joins sharply from the right.

Leave the pines behind and enter a shrubby area, where a fork awaits. Stay left and stroll through rolling and increasingly open terrain. The right-hand branch of the fork is parallel to, and about 40 feet right of, your trail. Several short connectors join the two trails, which are separated by a hedge of shrubs. From a low rise, enjoy views ahead and left of Miacomet Pond, a long, narrow body of water.

A rest bench offers a scenic perch just past the second connector to the neighboring trail. Soon the trails diverge; yours curves left and descends toward the pond through a corridor of shrubs. Just ahead is a four-way junction beside the pond. Here turn right on a grassy, possibly muddy, trail and go through a gap in an old fence, where closely spaced upright posts block vehicle access. Just before reaching the property boundary, marked by a chain between two posts, turn sharply right on a trail that climbs on a gentle grade.

Now follow the trail as it bends right (north) and eventually runs parallel to the trail you were on earlier, which is about 40 feet to the right. After the two parallel trails merge, bear left and retrace your route to the next junction. Here angle left through a corridor of shrubs; then curve right, into a clearing. Approaching a residential area, the trail bends sharply right. Make a winding descent amid pines and shrubs, and then rejoin the main trail. Bear left and retrace your route to the parking area.

GENERAL

DISTANCE 0.9 miles

TYPE OF WALK Balloon

DIFFICULTY Easy

TIME TO WALK 1 hour or less

MAPS *Nantucket*, USGS

SCENERY Forest, grassland, marsh

EXPOSURE TO SUN Partial

TRAIL TRAFFIC Light

TRAIL SURFACE(S) Dirt

TRAILS OPEN All year

FEES/PASSES None

FACILITIES None

TRAIL USE

BICYCLES Allowed

DOGS Allowed on leash

HUNTING Not allowed near houses (posted)

HEALTH STATS

NUMBER OF STEPS 2,250

ESTIMATED CALORIES BURNED 107

DIRECTIONS TO TRAILHEAD

From the intersection of Hummock Pond and Milk roads (southwest of Nantucket Town), take Hummock Pond Road southwest for 1.5 miles to a large, mowed-grass parking area on the right. The trailhead is on the northwest side of the parking area.

Forest, Meadow, and Marsh Meander

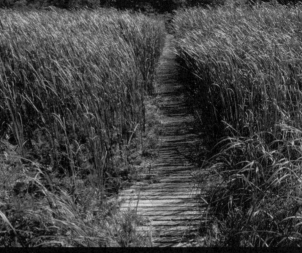

Boardwalk crosses freshwater wetland at Gardner proper

WALK SUMMARY

This easy walk leads visitors amid stands of tall pine trees, through a wildflower-filled meadow, and then, via a boardwalk, across a freshwater marsh filled with cattails and ferns. An osprey pole may hold an active nest and provide opportunities to view these magnificent raptors.

DESCRIPTION

From the trailhead, walk through a gap in a split-rail fence, pass a helpful map on a post, and angle left on a dirt path through an open field. After about 100 yards, a dirt road joins from the left. Go straight, now on a dirt road. Descend gently to merge with a dirt road that joins sharply from the left. Bear right and now follow the pine-bordered

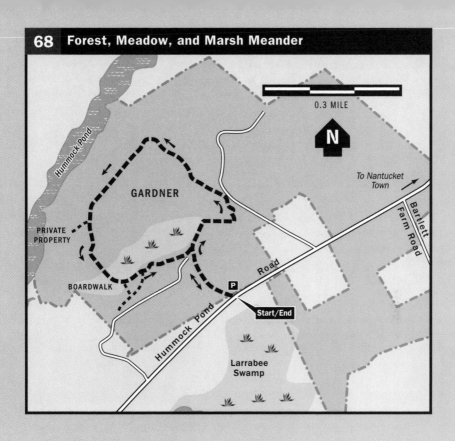

road as it makes a few sharply angled bends and reaches a four-way junction with another dirt road.

Veer left and enjoy a shady stroll amid stately pines. Soon reach a huge open field, on the right, which may be decorated with wildflowers in season. Now the road takes a sharp leftward bend; there is another map on a post here, and an osprey pole rises in the distance. More open fields await as the road heads southwest to a four-way junction beyond which is private property marked with a NO TRESPASSING sign.

Here turn left on a mowed path and skirt the west edge of an open field. The path curves right and comes to a boardwalk. Bear left to get on the boardwalk, which crosses an extensive cattail marsh. After the boardwalk ends, walk gently uphill on a dirt trail that leads into a pine forest.

About 150 feet from the end of the boardwalk, turn left on a mowed path that skirts the marsh, which is screened from view by a line of trees and shrubs to the left. Walk about 100 yards, and then merge with a faint track joining sharply on the right. Continue straight, soon entering a narrow corridor of

FLORA	FAUNA
Some of the tallest pitch pines on Nantucket, many with ropy vines of poison ivy clinging to their trunks, occupy parts of this 134-acre Nantucket Islands Land Bank property. Arrowwood, bayberry, bearberry, black cherry, and a fine array of wildflowers grow here as well. Cattails and ferns thrive in a lovely freshwater marsh.	A pair of nesting osprey, sometimes called fish hawks because of their seafood diet, may be using a nesting pole on the property.

shrubs and trees. In more open terrain, merge with a dirt road by angling left, and then close the loop at a junction 25 feet ahead. From here, turn right and retrace your route to the parking area.

Pond Promenade

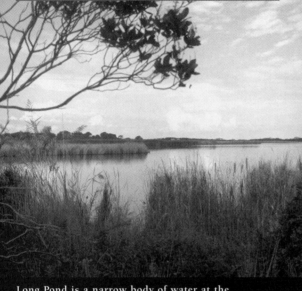

Long Pond is a narrow body of water at the west end of Nantucket.

WALK SUMMARY

This easy out-and-back stroll beside Long Pond explores part of a 64-acre property owned by the Nantucket Islands Land Bank. The various habitats—grassland, heathland, pond, shrubland, and wetland—along with the presence of an osprey pole, which may have an active nest, make this an ideal walk for birders and native-plant enthusiasts.

DESCRIPTION

From the trailhead, which is marked by a split-rail fence and a gate, follow a grassy, shrub-bordered path that leads along the southeast side of Long Pond. The opposite shore is lined with houses, dramatizing the value of preserving open space. An osprey pole ahead may be occupied by a nesting pair of the fish-eating

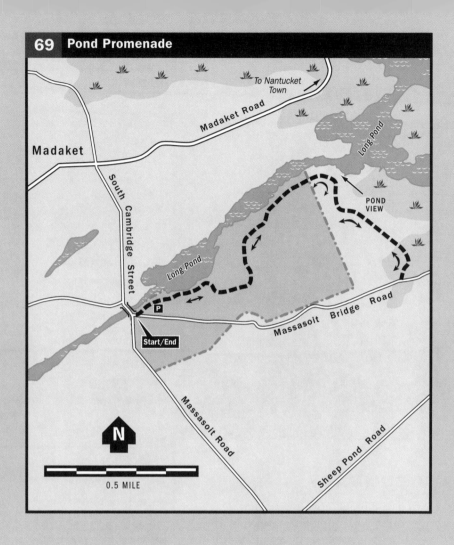

To Nantucket Town

Madaket Road

Madaket

Long Pond

South Cambridge Street

Long Pond

POND VIEW

P

Massasoit Bridge Road

Start/End

Massasoit Road

Sheep Pond Road

N

0.5 MILE

raptors, whose return from the DDT-caused brink of extinction is one of the great environmental success stories.

Another bird to look for here, although much more secretive and hard to find than the osprey, is the American bittern, a heronlike marsh dweller. Bitterns, colored to match the marsh grasses and reeds, hide themselves by adopting a rigid upright posture with bill held straight up. When this posture doesn't provide enough protection, the bird erupts in flight and flies low over the marsh to its next hiding spot.

Pass a trail, on the right, and stroll beside a sandy hillside carpeted with low-growing bearberry, where asters may be in bloom. Now wander through a corridor of shrubs and vines to a junction where the trail merges with a dirt

FLORA

Shrubs bordering the trail include black huckleberry, bayberry, chokeberry, scrub oak, sweet pepperbush, arrowwood, pasture rose, sheep laurel, winterberry, bearberry, highbush blueberry, and dwarf chestnut oak. Long Pond is fringed with common reed, or phragmites, which provides cover and nesting areas for birds but is considered an invasive nonnative species. A few trees—pitch pine, black cherry, shadbush—dot the otherwise open landscape, which in fall may be decorated with wildflowers, including asters and goldenrods. Greenbrier, wild grape, and Virginia creeper intertwine beside the trail.

FAUNA

Waterfowl, wading birds, raptors, and songbirds all live or visit here, making this trail a fine birding area. Eastern cottontails may be plentiful.

road that joins sharply from the right. Angle left onto the road and pass the osprey pole, which is left. The open, shrub-dotted terrain affords more views of Long Pond, which, true to its name, is a long, narrow body of water bordered by wetlands.

Now meet a short trail, on the left, which offers closer views of the pond. Beyond this junction, follow the dirt road as it curves right and climbs gently to a T-junction with another dirt road. From here, retrace your route to the parking area.

GENERAL

DISTANCE 1.7 miles

TYPE OF WALK Balloon

DIFFICULTY Moderate

TIME TO WALK 1 hour or less

MAPS *Visitor's Trail Guide to Squam Swamp*, Nantucket Conservation Foundation, Inc.; *Siasconset*, USGS

SCENERY Bog, forest, swamp, vernal pool

EXPOSURE TO SUN Partial

TRAIL TRAFFIC Light

TRAIL SURFACE(S) Dirt

TRAILS OPEN All year

FEES/PASSES None

FACILITIES None

TRAIL USE

BICYCLES Not allowed

DOGS Not allowed

HUNTING Allowed in season

HEALTH STATS

NUMBER OF STEPS 3,825

ESTIMATED CALORIES BURNED 182

DIRECTIONS TO TRAILHEAD

From the intersection of Polpis and Wauwinet roads (east of Nantucket Town), take Wauwinet Road north for 1.4 miles and turn right on a dirt road that goes about 100 feet to a large dirt parking area. The trailhead is on the north side of the parking area.

Squam Swamp Interpretive Trail

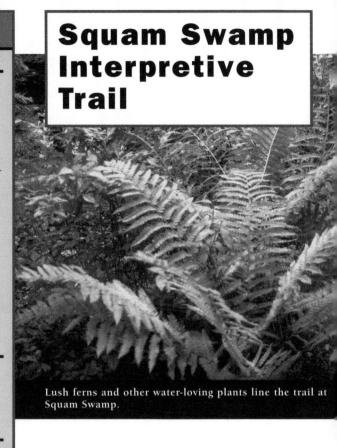

Lush ferns and other water-loving plants line the trail at Squam Swamp.

WALK SUMMARY

This easy, enjoyable ramble takes you through a red-maple-and-tupelo swamp, plus adjacent uplands, where plant enthusiasts will enjoy identifying native species and bird-watchers can hone their "birding by ear" skills.

Boldface numbers in the description below refer to numbered markers, most spaced approximately 100 feet apart along the trail, which are keyed to text in *Visitor's Trail Guide to Squam Swamp*, a pamphlet published by the Nantucket Conservation Foundation. There is a box for these brochures at the trailhead; please consider recycling the brochure by returning it to the box after your walk.

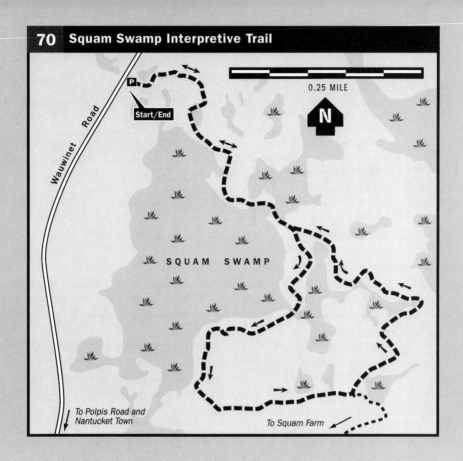

DESCRIPTION

From the trailhead, go through a gap in a split-rail fence and follow a sandy trail that descends gently into a red-maple-and-tupelo swamp. In fall, these two tree species provide a colorful display. The lush understory of dense shrubs and tall ferns creates a junglelike feeling. After several hundred feet, arrive at marker **1**, indicating the different vegetative communities found here. Bear right at a junction with a closed trail, on the left, and reach marker **2**, which highlights various species of oaks—white, black, scrub, and dwarf chestnut.

A level walk leads to marker **3**, indicating a hardwood forest, which is relatively rare on Nantucket. Curve right, then turn right to marker **4**, which indicates a partially uprooted red-maple tree. Now cross a seasonally wet area via wooden planks and come to markers **5**, for a nearby glacial boulder, and **6**, for a vernal pool. Marker **7** indicates an area of sphagnum beside the trail.

FLORA	FAUNA
Tupelo, red maple, white oak, black oak, hickory, sassafras, and American beech are some of the trees found in the swamp. Shrubs include arrowwood, sweet pepperbush, swamp azalea, highbush blueberry, dwarf chestnut oak, and bayberry. Poison ivy is present, along with grapevines. Early-spring wildflowers include Canada mayflower, wood anemone, starflower, and trailing arbutus. Goldenrods and asters add color in late summer and fall.	Blue jays, gray catbirds, downy woodpeckers, northern flickers, eastern towhees, yellow warblers, black-capped chickadees, great crested flycatchers, and red-tailed hawks are among the common birds found in the swamp.

Climb on a gentle grade to a rest bench and marker **8,** for areas of higher elevation that rise out of the swamp. Turn right and descend to marker **9,** indicating a seasonal pool that provides habitat for spotted turtles, state-listed as a species of special concern. Now the route angles left, then swings left and passes marker **10,** for soil moisture. Climb over a low rise to marker **11,** for red maples, which in a swamp may grow to 100 feet tall and live nearly a century. A winding course leads to marker **12,** for one of Nantucket's few flowing streams.

Turn left and cross a wooden bridge to marker **13,** for stream water colored brown by tannins released from decaying vegetation. Turn left and go about 100 feet to marker **14,** for a stand of tupelo, or black gum, trees. Now pass the returning leg of the self-guided trail, which is on the left. Marker **15** indicates mockernut, a type of hickory, which is not very common on Nantucket but is locally abundant on Cape Cod. "Leaflets three, let it be" is the rule for poison ivy at marker **16.** Now the trail curves right. Marker **17** is for lichens, which are actually two plants, an algae and a fungus, living in close association. Now climb a low rise to marker **18,** for more lichens. Curve left and walk about 100 feet to marker **19,** for this glacially formed hilltop and a rest bench.

From here, descend to marker **20,** which highlights moss-shrouded trees. A narrow and winding but mostly level trail leads through the dense understory to a boardwalk and then wooden planks over a seasonally wet area. Marker **21** indicates a fallen red maple. Ahead, another red maple's outstretched limbs reach across the trail. Pass marker **22,** for a vernal pool, and climb to marker **23,** which indicates highbush blueberry. Another tall shrub, bayberry, is at marker **24.**

Now follow a curvy, rolling course about 200 feet to marker **25,** for a "hidden forest." Bear left and enter a magical grove of American beech trees, venerable giants with branching limbs and partially exposed roots that crisscross the trail. Marker **26** nearby is for fox grape, a type of wild grape. The large trees here block most of the light, resulting in a lack of shrubs in the understory as indicated by marker **27.** Marker **28** is for a large American beech.

Now begin a snaking ascent, passing marker **29,** for tupelo, or black gum. Emerge from dense forest into a sunnier realm, where marker **30** indicates an unusually tall (10- to 15-foot) scrub oak. Enjoy a level ramble past markers **31,** for red maple, and **32,** for black cherry. In a small clearing, a rest bench awaits opposite marker **33,** for a lack of mature trees. A tunnel of shrubs and vines, including poison ivy, leads to marker **34,** for northern arrowwood, a species of viburnum.

Wind downhill to maker **35,** which indicates beaked hazelnut, a shrub that produces edible fruits enjoyed by birds and small mammals. After losing more elevation, the trail finds level ground near maker **36,** for distinct layers of vegetation in the forest. Marker **37,** in a low-lying area, is for the surrounding fern garden. From here, angle slightly right and climb to marker **38,** for more American beech trees.

About 50 feet ahead is a fork and a trail post with an arrow pointing left (the trail going right leads to the Nantucket Conservation Foundation's 210-acre Squam Farm property, which also has walking trails.) Bear left at the fork; then wind along to marker **39,** for American holly. Marker **40,** just ahead, indicates a sphagnum bog. Walk on level ground to marker **41,** for sweet pepperbush, whose fragrance permeates the forest in midsummer.

Now arrive at a little clearing and a T-junction. A rest bench is right and marker **42,** for upland plants, is across the junction. Turn left and pass marker **43,** for sassafras, a tree with mitten-shaped leaves. Now the trail bends left and comes to a trail post with an arrow pointing right. Turn sharply right, descend slightly, and then, at marker **44,** pass two different trees—a red maple and a tupelo—that appear to be fused together.

About 50 feet ahead, angle right and cross a seasonally wet area via a boardwalk. Now the trail curves left and passes a few large holly trees, marker **45.** A winding ascent leads to marker **46,** for swamp azalea. Just beyond a beautiful red-maple tree hung with grape vines, cross another boardwalk and curve left to marker **47,** for mockernut hickory. Follow the trail as it swings left and enters a more open area, where goldenrod, a bee favorite, blooms in late summer and fall. Marker **48** indicates more fox grape.

Amble through a parklike forest to marker **49,** for greenbrier. Marker **50** indicates a place where the fallen part of a beech tree has opened the forest canopy, providing light for other plants to thrive. Walk about 100 feet to where an arrow on a trail post points left, and heed its advice. A vernal pool, marker **51,** is just ahead. A gently rolling course leads past the fallen trunk of an American beech, marker **52.**

Soon stroll by tall ropy grape vines, which drape over tree limbs and hang down to the trail. Marker **53** indicates early-spring wildflowers, which bloom briefly on forest floor. Marker **54** is for shadbush, a smooth-barked tree with oval, finely toothed leaves. At a T-junction just ahead, turn right and retrace your route to the trailhead.

Barn and Back

GENERAL

DISTANCE 3.4 miles

TYPE OF WALK Balloon

DIFFICULTY Moderate

TIME TO WALK 2–3 hours

MAPS *Information and Map for Visitors to The Sanford Farm, Ram Pasture, and The Woods,* Nantucket Conservation Foundation, Inc.; *Nantucket,* USGS

SCENERY Atlantic Ocean, grassland, shrubland, pond

EXPOSURE TO SUN Full

TRAIL TRAFFIC Heavy

TRAIL SURFACE(S) Dirt

TRAILS OPEN All year

FEES/PASSES None

FACILITIES None

TRAIL USE

BICYCLES Allowed only on established trails

DOGS Allowed on leash

HUNTING Not allowed

HEALTH STATS

NUMBER OF STEPS 7,650

ESTIMATED CALORIES BURNED 364

DIRECTIONS TO TRAILHEAD

From the intersection of Cliff and Madaket roads (west of Nantucket Town), take Madaket Road east for 0.1 mile to a large dirt parking area on the right (south) side of the road, beside the bike path. The trailhead is on the south-east corner of the parking area.

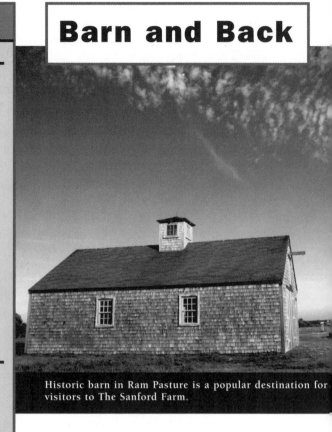

Historic barn in Ram Pasture is a popular destination for visitors to The Sanford Farm.

WALK SUMMARY

This enjoyable excursion traverses a former farm and grazing area wedged between Trots Swamp and Hummock Pond, southwest of Nantucket Town. The habitats include grassland, shrubland, a pine grove, and a glacially formed freshwater pond. Before the arrival of Europeans, the area had a long history of use by Native Americans. After settlement, sheep and other livestock kept the grasslands open, but today's land managers for the Nantucket Conservation Foundation preserve precious sandplain habitats through the use of mowing and prescribed burning. Boldface numbers in the description refer to numbered interpretive markers beside the trail. Please stay on established roadways and trails.

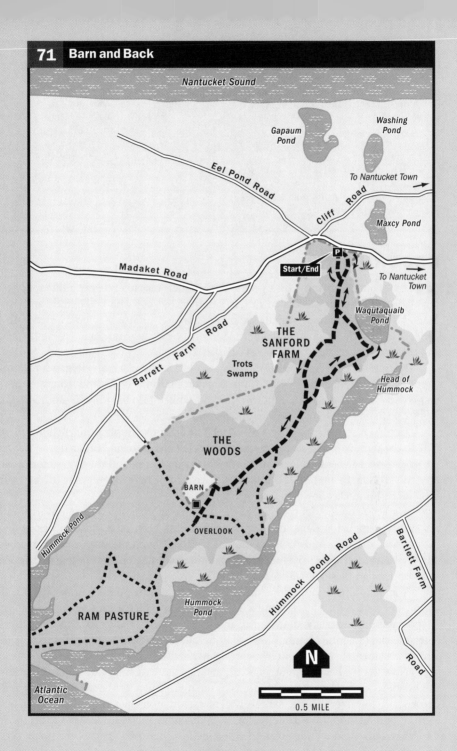

Nantucket Sound

Gapaum
Pond

Washing
Pond

Eel Pond Road

To Nantucket Town

Cliff Road

Maxcy Pond

P

Start/End

Madaket Road

To Nantucket
Town

Waqutaquaib
Pond

THE
SANFORD
FARM

Barrett Farm Road

Trots
Swamp

Head of
Hummock

THE
WOODS

BARN

OVERLOOK

Hummock Pond

Hummock Pond Road

Bartlett Farm

RAM PASTURE

Hummock
Pond

Road

N

0.5 MILE

Atlantic
Ocean

FLORA	FAUNA
Wildflowers in the grasslands provide splashes of color, as do vines such as Virginia creeper, wild grape, greenbrier, and poison ivy in the fall. Arrowwood, bearberry, bayberry, scrub oak, sweet pepperbush, highbush blueberry, black huckleberry, sheep laurel, and groundsel tree thrive in the sandplain habitat, beside Trots Swamp, and near Hummock Pond, which is fringed with cattails and common reed. Pitch pine, black cherry, shadbush, and hawthorn are among the trees found here.	Waterfowl, fish, and turtles are at home on and in Hummock Pond. Overhead, look for gulls, crows, and raptors, including osprey, northern harriers, and red-tailed hawks. Short-eared owls, state-listed as endangered, have been spotted here, as well as northern harriers, state-listed as threatened.

DESCRIPTION

From the trailhead, marked by a gate and a wooden turnstile, follow a dirt road south through open country decorated in late summer and fall with goldenrods and asters. Marker **1,** which indicates Waqutaquaib Pond, whose surface may be covered with lily pads, is to the left. Soon an alternate trail from the parking area joins on the right (you will use this trail on the return to visit marker **2**).

A depression in the land on the right, marker **3,** is the site of a former farm, which operated here through the 1920s. A junction and marker **4** (grassland management) are just ahead. Land managers use mowing and prescribed burning to keep sandplain grasslands open and free from encroaching trees and shrubs.

Continue straight, passing a rest bench and a grove of pitch pines, both on your left. To the right is Trots Swamp, marker **5,** a freshwater wetland bordered by a rich variety of shrubs. The Sanford Farm property ends at marker **6,** and the road enters a property called Ram Pasture and The Woods. Views from here extend east to the church steeples of Nantucket Town.

Marker **7,** on the right, describes the prior use of the property as a private hunting reserve. The trail that departed at marker **4** rejoins here, at a junction beside a rest bench. At about the 1-mile point, a mowed path shown on the map as a dirt road goes sharply right, and about 50 feet ahead, another one not on the map goes left. Walk straight through these junctions and enter The Woods, marker **14.**

Wander through a corridor of dense shrubs and trees, passing marker **15.** The thorny tree here is hawthorn, about a dozen species of which are found on the Cape and Islands, although rarely widespread or in great numbers. Marker **16,** on the left, indicates the site of a former farm. These sites are often identified by plantings of fruit trees and/or ornamental shrubs, and by depressions that were once cellar holes.

Now the road curves right, jogs left, and reaches a clearing with a dramatic view of the Atlantic Ocean. A photogenic barn is to the right, and a rest bench is left. The widest expanse of Hummock Pond, whose waters extend from just behind a barrier beach fronting the Atlantic to near the trailhead, is downhill and left. Marker **17,** on the left, describes a dike and a bridge that once spanned the narrowest part of the pond.

Immediately ahead is a four-way junction where a mowed path, shown on the map as a dirt road, crosses your road. Just beyond the junction is Ram Pasture Overlook, marker **18.** After enjoying this beautiful spot, retrace your route to the junction at marker **7** and veer right on a dirt road. Marker **8,** on the left, describes the two types of ticks commonly found on Nantucket.

The road curves right and traverses open terrain dotted with low shrubs. An osprey pole, ahead, may be in use by a nesting pair of these fish-eating raptors saved from extinction by the banning of DDT. A short trail, on the right, leads to marker **9,** beside Hummock Pond. Back on the dirt road, marker **10** describes evidence of Native American settlements nearby. Climb on a gentle grade and curve left to a rest bench and marker **11,** both on the left.

Walk about 150 feet ahead to a bluff, marker **12,** overlooking Head of Hummock Pond, a glacial kettle pond. A cattail-choked channel connects Head of Hummock Pond with Hummock Pond. Now the road bends left and descends gently toward a grove of pitch pines, marker **13.** Pines of various species, along with hardwoods, were planted on the Cape and Islands to help control erosion caused by decades of cutting and clearing.

Emerge from the pine grove and in several hundred feet merge with the other branch of the trail at marker **4.** From here, retrace your route to the junction near marker **1.** Now veer left on a single-track trail and climb a grassy hillside to the Sanford Farm Overlook, marker **2.** From here, follow the trail north and descend to the parking area.

GENERAL

DISTANCE 1 mile

TYPE OF WALK Balloon

DIFFICULTY Easy

TIME TO WALK 1 hour or less

MAPS *Information for Visitors to the Tupancy Links,* Nantucket Conservation Foundation, Inc.; *Nantucket,* USGS

SCENERY Grassland, heathland, Nantucket Sound

EXPOSURE TO SUN Full

TRAIL TRAFFIC Moderate

TRAIL SURFACE(S) Dirt, grass, sand, wood chips

TRAILS OPEN All year

FEES/PASSES None

FACILITIES None

TRAIL USE

BICYCLES Not allowed

DOGS Allowed on leash

HUNTING Not allowed

HEALTH STATS

NUMBER OF STEPS 2,250

ESTIMATED CALORIES BURNED 107

DIRECTIONS TO TRAILHEAD

From the intersection of Cliff Road and Easton Street in Nantucket Town, take Cliff Road northwest, then southwest, for 1.3 miles to a dirt-and-gravel parking area on the right, beside the bike path. The trailhead is on the north side of the parking area, at a turnstile.

Note: The Nantucket Conservation Foundation office, where maps and other information are available, is at 118 Cliff Road, about 1 mile from its intersection with Easton Street.

A Link to the Past

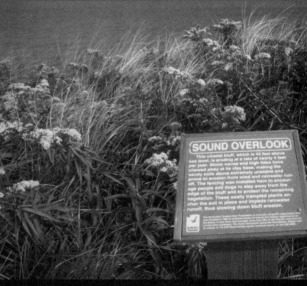

Trail at Tupancy Links leads to an overlook of Nantucket Sound.

WALK SUMMARY

Step back in time by strolling through this former golf course, donated by its former owners to the Nantucket Conservation Foundation. Tupancy Links contains fine examples of sandplain habitats, including grasslands and heathlands. The high point of the walk, literally and figuratively, is the Nantucket Sound overlook, a favorite sunset-watching spot featuring 360-degree views.

DESCRIPTION

From the trailhead, pass through a turnstile and then walk on a wood-chip path that angles left and climbs on a gentle grade. Arrive at a fork, bear right, and enjoy ever-improving views eastward to Nantucket Town, where church steeples rise over picturesque homes. Soon the trail reaches what used

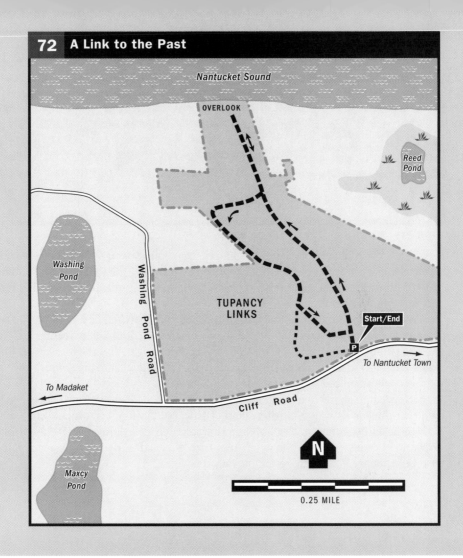

Nantucket Sound

OVERLOOK

Reed Pond

Washing Pond

Washing Pond Road

TUPANCY LINKS

Start/End

P

To Nantucket Town

To Madaket

Cliff Road

Maxcy Pond

N

0.25 MILE

to be a putting green on a golf course that operated here from 1921 until 1953. The property was donated to the Foundation by the course's former owners, Oswald A. (Tup) Tupancy, a golf pro, and his wife, Sallie Gail Harris Tupancy, who served on the Foundation's board of trustees.

Bear left and head northwest, following a path worn in the grass through a shallow swale. After about 100 yards, pass an interpretive sign describing the discovery in 1909 of Nantucket shadbush, a rare plant of the northern Atlantic coast. Nearby homes serve as a reminder, if one is needed, of the value of preserving open space.

Angle right at a fork and walk on a sandy path that soon changes to wood chips and climbs gently to a fenced cliff edge overlooking Nantucket Sound.

Several rest benches are here. From this fine vantage point, about 40 feet above sea level, views extend east to Coatue Point and the jetties guarding the entrance to Nantucket Harbor; northeast to the lighthouse at Great Point; and west to Dionis Beach, Eel Point, and Tuckernuck Island.

When ready, retrace your route to the previous junction and bear right. Walk about 150 feet to a fork, angle left, and immediately merge with a dirt road by veering left. Now descend gently beside a split-rail fence, which is on the right, and the former golf links, which are left. A nearby interpretive sign describes the dune landscape, which over the years became stabilized by grasses, vines, and shrubs.

Now climb gently to a junction and leave the dirt road by swinging left on a sandy path that threads its way through a stand of Japanese black pines, which were planted on Nantucket beginning in the 1890s but became infested during the 1940s by black turpentine beetles. Many of the older trees here are dead or dying. Soon reach a fork; from here, retrace your route to the parking area.

Walking
Cape
Islands

a comprehensive guide to
the walking and hiking trails
of Cape Cod, Martha's Vineyard,
and Nantucket

APPENDIX A: BEST WALKS

APPENDIX A: BEST WALKS

▶ **MODERATE WALKS (1 to 5 miles with some hills)**

CAPE COD: UPPER CAPE

Walk 1: Bourne, Four Ponds Conservation Area
Walk 3: Sandwich, Maple Swamp Conservation Lands
Walk 7: Falmouth, Falmouth Town Forest
Walk 8: Mashpee, Lowell Holly Reservation
Walk 9: Mashpee, Mashpee River Woodlands
Walk 11: Mashpee, South Mashpee Pine Barrens Conservation Area

CAPE COD: MID-CAPE

Walk 13: Barnstable, Old Jail Lane Conservation Area
Walk 15: Barnstable, West Barnstable Conservation Area
Walk 16: Yarmouth, Callery-Darling Conservation Area

CAPE COD: LOWER CAPE

Walk 21: Brewster, Nickerson State Park, Cliff and Little Cliff Ponds
Walk 22: Brewster, Nickerson State Park, Silas Road
Walk 23: Brewster, Punkhorn Parklands, Calf Field Pond
Walk 27: Harwich, Hawksnest State Park

CAPE COD: OUTER CAPE

Walk 31: Eastham, Cape Cod National Seashore, Nauset Marsh Trail and Coast Guard Beach
Walk 32: Eastham, Cape Cod National Seashore, Red Maple Swamp and Fort Hill
Walk 35: Wellfleet, Cape Cod National Seashore, Wellfleet and Truro Ponds
Walk 36: Wellfleet, Wellfleet Bay Wildlife Sanctuary (Mass Audubon), Bay View Trail and
    Fresh Brook Pathway
Walk 38: Truro, Cape Cod National Seashore, North Pamet Area, Bearberry Hill and Bog House
Walk 39: Truro, Cape Cod National Seashore, North Pamet Area, Truro Hills

MARTHA'S VINEYARD

Walk 45: Chilmark, Fulling Mill Brook Preserve
Walk 47: Chilmark, Menemsha Hills Reservation
Walk 48: Chilmark, Middle Road Sanctuary
Walk 49: Chilmark, Peaked Hill Reservation
Walk 50: Chilmark, Waskosim's Rock Reservation
Walk 51: West Tisbury, Cedar Tree Neck Sanctuary
Walk 52: West Tisbury, Long Point Wildlife Refuge
Walk 53: West Tisbury, Manuel F. Correllus State Forest
Walk 54: West Tisbury, Sepiessa Point Reservation
Walk 58: Oak Bluffs, Trade Wind Fields and Farm Pond Preserves
Walk 62: Edgartown, Manuel F. Correllus State Forest
Walk 63: Edgartown, Chappaquiddick Island, Poucha Pond Reservation
Walk 65: Edgartown, Chappaquiddick Island, Wasque Reservation

APPENDIX A: BEST WALKS

▶ MODERATE WALKS (continued)

NANTUCKET

Walk 66: Nantucket, Altar Rock

Walk 70: Nantucket, Squam Swamp

Walk 71: Nantucket, The Sanford Farm, Ram Pasture, and The Woods

▶ DIFFICULT WALKS (more than 5 miles)

CAPE COD: MID-CAPE

Walk 14: Barnstable, Sandy Neck

CAPE COD: LOWER CAPE

Walk 25: Brewster, Punkhorn Parklands, Grand Tour

CAPE COD: OUTER CAPE

Walk 34: Wellfleet, Cape Cod National Seashore, Great Island Trail

Walk 43: Provincetown, Cape Cod National Seashore, Long Point

Walk 44: Provincetown, Cape Cod National Seashore, Race Point and Hatches Harbor

▶ WALKS WHERE DOGS ARE NOT ALLOWED

Walk 5: Falmouth, Ashumet Holly Wildlife Sanctuary (Mass Audubon)

Walk 31: Eastham, Cape Cod National Seashore, Nauset Marsh Trail and Coast Guard Beach

Walk 32: Eastham, Cape Cod National Seashore, Red Maple Swamp and Fort Hill

Walk 33: Wellfleet, Cape Cod National Seashore, Atlantic White Cedar Swamp Trail

Walk 34: Wellfleet, Cape Cod National Seashore, Great Island Trail

Walk 36: Wellfleet, Wellfleet Bay Wildlife Sanctuary (Mass Audubon), Bay View Trail and
Fresh Brook Pathway

Walk 37: Wellfleet, Wellfleet Bay Wildlife Sanctuary (Mass Audubon), Goose Pond Trail

Walk 40: Truro, Cape Cod National Seashore, Pilgrim Spring Area, Pilgrim Spring Trail

Walk 41: Truro, Cape Cod National Seashore, Pilgrim Spring Area, Small's Swamp Trail

Walk 42: Provincetown, Cape Cod National Seashore, Beech Forest Trail

Walk 44: Provincetown, Cape Cod National Seashore, Race Point and Hatches Harbor
(May 1–October 1)

Walk 47: Chilmark, Menemsha Hills Reservation

Walk 52: West Tisbury, Long Point Wildlife Refuge

Walk 60: Edgartown, Felix Neck Wildlife Sanctuary (Mass Audubon), Jessica Hancock Trail

Walk 61: Edgartown, Felix Neck Wildlife Sanctuary (Mass Audubon), Woodland Wonderland

Walk 70: Nantucket, Squam Swamp, Squam Swamp Interpretive Trail

▶ WALKS WHERE HUNTING IS NOT ALLOWED

Walk 5: Falmouth, Ashumet Holly Wildlife Sanctuary (Mass Audubon)

Walk 6: Falmouth, Beebe Woods

Walk 8: Mashpee, Lowell Holly Reservation

Walk 9: Mashpee, Mashpee River Woodlands

APPENDIX A: BEST WALKS

Walk 11: Mashpee, South Mashpee Pine Barrens Conservation Area
Walk 17: Yarmouth, Historical Society of Old Yarmouth
Walk 20: Brewster, Cape Cod Museum of Natural History
Walk 21: Brewster, Nickerson State Park, Cliff and Little Cliff Ponds
Walk 22: Brewster, Nickerson State Park, Silas Road
Walk 23: Brewster, Punkhorn Parklands, Calf Field Pond
Walk 24: Brewster, Punkhorn Parklands, Eagle Point
Walk 25: Brewster, Punkhorn Parklands, Grand Tour
Walk 28: Chatham, Monomoy National Wildlife Refuge (not allowed from land; allowed in season from boat)
Walk 29: Orleans, Kent's Point Conservation Area
Walk 30: Orleans, Paw Wah Pond Conservation Area
Walk 31: Eastham, Cape Cod National Seashore, Nauset Marsh Trail and Coast Guard Beach
Walk 32: Eastham, Cape Cod National Seashore, Red Maple Swamp and Fort Hill
Walk 33: Wellfleet, Cape Cod National Seashore, Atlantic White Cedar Swamp Trail
Walk 34: Wellfleet, Cape Cod National Seashore, Great Island Trail
Walk 35: Wellfleet, Cape Cod National Seashore, Wellfleet and Truro Ponds
Walk 36: Wellfleet, Wellfleet Bay Wildlife Sanctuary (Mass Audubon), Bay View Trail and Fresh Brook Pathway
Walk 37: Wellfleet, Wellfleet Bay Wildlife Sanctuary (Mass Audubon), Goose Pond Trail
Walk 38: Truro, Cape Cod National Seashore, North Pamet Area, Bearberry Hill and Bog House
Walk 39: Truro, Cape Cod National Seashore, North Pamet Area, Truro Hills
Walk 40: Truro, Cape Cod National Seashore, Pilgrim Spring Area, Pilgrim Spring Trail
Walk 41: Truro, Cape Cod National Seashore, Pilgrim Spring Area, Small's Swamp Trail
Walk 42: Provincetown, Cape Cod National Seashore, Beech Forest Trail
Walk 43: Provincetown, Cape Cod National Seashore, Long Point
Walk 44: Provincetown, Cape Cod National Seashore, Race Point and Hatches Harbor
Walk 47: Chilmark, Menemsha Hills Reservation
Walk 48: Chilmark, Middle Road Sanctuary
Walk 51: West Tisbury, Cedar Tree Neck Sanctuary
Walk 57: Tisbury, West Chop Woods
Walk 58: Oak Bluffs, Trade Wind Fields and Farm Pond Preserves
Walk 59: Edgartown, Caroline Tuthill Preserve
Walk 60: Edgartown, Felix Neck Wildlife Sanctuary (Mass Audubon), Jessica Hancock Trail
Walk 61: Edgartown, Felix Neck Wildlife Sanctuary (Mass Audubon), Woodland Wonderland
Walk 65: Edgartown, Chappaquiddick Island, Wasque Reservation
Walk 67: Nantucket, Burchell
Walk 68: Nantucket, Gardner
Walk 71: Nantucket, The Sanford Farm, Ram Pasture, and The Woods
Walk 72: Nantucket, Tupancy Links

▶ BEST BIRDING WALKS

Walk 1: Bourne, Four Ponds Conservation Area
Walk 5: Falmouth, Ashumet Holly Wildlife Sanctuary (Mass Audubon)

APPENDIX A: BEST WALKS

▶ BEST BIRDING WALKS (continued)

Walk 14: Barnstable, Sandy Neck
Walk 23: Brewster, Punkhorn Parklands, Calf Field Pond
Walk 24: Brewster, Punkhorn Parklands, Eagle Point
Walk 25: Brewster, Punkhorn Parklands, Grand Tour
Walk 28: Chatham, Monomoy National Wildlife Refuge
Walk 31: Eastham, Cape Cod National Seashore, Nauset Marsh Trail and Coast Guard Beach
Walk 32: Eastham, Cape Cod National Seashore, Red Maple Swamp and Fort Hill
Walk 37: Wellfleet, Wellfleet Bay Wildlife Sanctuary (Mass Audubon), Goose Pond Trail
Walk 42: Provincetown, Cape Cod National Seashore, Beech Forest Trail
Walk 44: Provincetown, Cape Cod National Seashore, Race Point and Hatches Harbor
Walk 45: Chilmark, Fulling Mill Brook Preserve
Walk 50: Chilmark, Waskosim's Rock Reservation
Walk 58: Oak Bluffs, Trade Wind Fields and Farm Pond Preserves
Walk 61: Edgartown, Felix Neck Wildlife Sanctuary (Mass Audubon), Woodland Wonderland
Walk 63: Edgartown, Chappaquiddick Island, Poucha Pond Reservation
Walk 66: Nantucket, Altar Rock
Walk 70: Nantucket, Squam Swamp, Squam Swamp Interpretive Trail

▶ BEST NATURE WALKS

Walk 5: Falmouth, Ashumet Holly Wildlife Sanctuary (Mass Audubon)
Walk 9: Mashpee, Mashpee River Woodlands
Walk 17: Yarmouth, Historical Society of Old Yarmouth
Walk 20: Brewster, Cape Cod Museum of Natural History
Walk 28: Chatham, Monomoy National Wildlife Refuge
Walk 31: Eastham, Cape Cod National Seashore, Nauset Marsh Trail and Coast Guard Beach
Walk 32: Eastham, Cape Cod National Seashore, Red Maple Swamp and Fort Hill
Walk 33: Wellfleet, Cape Cod National Seashore, Atlantic White Cedar Swamp Trail
Walk 36: Wellfleet, Wellfleet Bay Wildlife Sanctuary (Mass Audubon), Bay View Trail and
 Fresh Brook Pathway
Walk 37: Wellfleet, Wellfleet Bay Wildlife Sanctuary (Mass Audubon), Goose Pond Trail
Walk 42: Provincetown, Cape Cod National Seashore, Beech Forest Trail
Walk 59: Edgartown, Caroline Tuthill Preserve
Walk 60: Edgartown, Felix Neck Wildlife Sanctuary (Mass Audubon), Jessica Hancock Trail
Walk 61: Edgartown, Felix Neck Wildlife Sanctuary (Mass Audubon), Woodland Wonderland
Walk 70: Nantucket, Squam Swamp
Walk 71: Nantucket, The Sanford Farm, Ram Pasture, and The Woods

▶ BEST OFF-SEASON WALKS

Walk 14: Barnstable, Sandy Neck
Walk 21: Brewster, Nickerson State Park, Cliff and Little Cliff Ponds
Walk 34: Wellfleet, Cape Cod National Seashore, Great Island Trail

APPENDIX A: BEST WALKS

Walk 35: Wellfleet, Cape Cod National Seashore, Wellfleet and Truro Ponds

Walk 43: Provincetown, Cape Cod National Seashore, Long Point

Walk 44: Provincetown, Cape Cod National Seashore, Race Point and Hatches Harbor

Walk 63: Edgartown, Chappaquiddick Island, Poucha Pond Reservation

Walk 65: Edgartown, Chappaquiddick Island, Wasque Reservation

Walk 66: Nantucket, Altar Rock

▶ BEST SCENIC VISTAS

Walk 9: Mashpee, Mashpee River Woodlands

Walk 14: Barnstable, Sandy Neck

Walk 18: Dennis, Crowes Pasture

Walk 28: Chatham, Monomoy National Wildlife Refuge

Walk 29: Orleans, Kent's Point Conservation Area

Walk 31: Eastham, Cape Cod National Seashore, Nauset Marsh Trail and Coast Guard Beach

Walk 34: Wellfleet, Cape Cod National Seashore, Great Island Trail

Walk 36: Wellfleet, Wellfleet Bay Wildlife Sanctuary (Mass Audubon), Bay View Trail and
Fresh Brook Pathway

Walk 38: Truro, Cape Cod National Seashore, North Pamet Area, Bearberry Hill and Bog House

Walk 39: Truro, Cape Cod National Seashore, North Pamet Area, Truro Hills

Walk 43: Provincetown, Cape Cod National Seashore, Long Point

Walk 44: Provincetown, Cape Cod National Seashore, Race Point and Hatches Harbor

Walk 46: Chilmark, Great Rock Bight Preserve

Walk 47: Chilmark, Menemsha Hills Reservation

Walk 51: West Tisbury, Cedar Tree Neck Sanctuary

Walk 52: West Tisbury, Long Point Wildlife Refuge

Walk 65: Edgartown, Chappaquiddick Island, Wasque Reservation

Walk 66: Nantucket, Altar Rock

Walk 71: Nantucket, The Sanford Farm, Ram Pasture, and The Woods

Walk 72: Nantucket, Tupancy Links

▶ BEST WALKS WITH CHILDREN
(nature/visitor center available)

Walk 20: Brewster, Cape Cod Museum of Natural History

Walk 31: Eastham, Cape Cod National Seashore, Nauset Marsh Trail and Coast Guard Beach
(omit out-and-back leg to Coast Guard Beach for a shorter loop walk)

Walk 37: Wellfleet, Wellfleet Bay Wildlife Sanctuary (Mass Audubon), Goose Pond Trail

Walk 60: Edgartown, Felix Neck Wildlife Sanctuary (Mass Audubon), Jessica Hancock Trail

Walk 61: Edgartown, Felix Neck Wildlife Sanctuary (Mass Audubon), Woodland Wonderland

▶ BEST WILDFLOWERS

Walk 5: Falmouth, Ashumet Holly Wildlife Sanctuary (Mass Audubon)

Walk 12: Barnstable, Bridge Creek Conservation Area

APPENDIX A: BEST WALKS

▶ BEST WILDFLOWERS (continued)

Walk 18: Dennis, Crowes Pasture

Walk 32: Eastham, Cape Cod National Seashore, Red Maple Swamp and Fort Hill

Walk 36: Wellfleet, Wellfleet Bay Wildlife Sanctuary (Mass Audubon), Bay View Trail and Fresh Brook Pathway

Walk 37: Wellfleet, Wellfleet Bay Wildlife Sanctuary (Mass Audubon), Goose Pond Trail

Walk 39: Truro, Cape Cod National Seashore, North Pamet Area, Truro Hills

Walk 49: Chilmark, Peaked Hill Reservation

Walk 51: West Tisbury, Cedar Tree Neck Sanctuary

Walk 53: West Tisbury, Manuel F. Correllus State Forest

Walk 54: West Tisbury, Sepiessa Point Reservation

Walk 55: Tisbury, Ripley's Field Preserve

Walk 62: Edgartown, Manuel F. Correllus State Forest

Walk 65: Edgartown, Chappaquiddick Island, Wasque Reservation

Walk 66: Nantucket, Altar Rock

Walk 68: Nantucket, Gardner

Walk 70: Nantucket, Squam Swamp

APPENDIX B:
RECOMMENDED READING

▶ CAPE COD

Beston, Henry. *The Outermost House*. New York: Henry Holt and Company, 1992.

Finch, Robert. *Cape Cod: Its Natural and Cultural History*. Washington, DC: National Park Service, 1993.

Finch, Robert. *Common Ground*. Boston: David R. Godine, 1981.

Finch, Robert. *Death of a Hornet*. Washington, DC: Counterpoint Press, 2000.

Grant, Kim. *Cape Cod, Martha's Vineyard & Nantucket: An Explorer's Guide,* 6th ed. Woodstock, VT: The Countryman Press, 2005.

Hay, John. *The Great Beach*. New York: W. W. Norton & Company, 1980.

Kittredge, Henry C. *Cape Cod: Its People and Their History,* 2nd ed. Hyannis, MA: Parnassus Imprints, Inc., 1987.

O'Connell, James C. *Becoming Cape Cod*. Lebanon, NH: University Press of New England, 2003.

Richardson, Wyman. *The House on Nauset Marsh*. Woodstock, VT: The Countryman Press, 1997.

Sabin, Shirley C. and Michael E. Whatley, eds. *Visitor's Guide to Cape Cod National Seashore*. Eastern National, 1999.

Schneider, Paul. *The Enduring Shore*. New York: Henry Holt and Company, 2000.

Thoreau, Henry D. *Cape Cod*. Orleans, MA: Parnassus Imprints, 1984.

Weintraub, David. *Adventure Kayaking: Cape Cod and Martha's Vineyard,* 2nd ed. Berkeley, CA: Wilderness Press, 2001.

▶ NATURAL HISTORY

Berrill, Michael and Deborah Berrill. *The North Atlantic Coast*. San Francisco: Sierra Club Books, 1981.

Buckley, Ann and Theodore O. Hendrickson. *Native Trees, Shrubs, and Woody Vines of Cape Cod and the Islands*. Dartmouth: University of Massachusetts, 1996.

Burt, William H. and Richard P. Grossenheider. *A Field Guide to the Mammals,* 3rd ed. New York: Houghton Mifflin Company, 1980.

Cape Cod Bird Club & Massachusetts Audubon Society. *Birding Cape Cod,* revised ed. Yarmouthport, MA: On Cape Publications, 2005.

Conant, Roger and Joseph T. Collins. *A Field Guide to Reptiles and Amphibians of Eastern and Central North America*. 3rd ed. expanded. New York: Houghton Mifflin Company, 1998.

DeGraaf, Richard M. and Mariko Yamasaki. *New England Wildlife*. Hanover, NH: University Press of New England, 2001.

Dickenson, Mary B., ed. *Field Guide to the Birds of North America,* 4th ed. Washington, DC: National Geographic Society, 1999.

APPENDIX B: RECOMMENDED READING

▶ NATURAL HISTORY (continued)

Drummon, Roger. *Ticks and What You Can Do about Them,* 3rd ed. Berkeley, CA: Wilderness Press, 2004.

Jorgensen, Neil. *Southern New England.* San Francisco: Sierra Club Books, 1978.

Little, Elbert L. *National Audubon Society Field Guide to North American Trees, Eastern Region.* New York: Alfred A. Knopf, 1997.

Newcomb, Lawrence. *Newcomb's Wildflower Guide.* Boston: Little, Brown and Company, 1977.

Oldale, Robert N. *Cape Cod, Martha's Vineyard & Nantucket: The Geologic Story,* revised ed. Yarmouthport, MA: On Cape Publications, 2001.

Petry, Loren C. and Marcia G. Norman. *A Beachcomber's Botany.* Chatham, MA: The Chatham Conservation Foundation, 1968.

Sibley, David Allen. *The Sibley Field Guide to Birds of Eastern North America.* New York: Alfred A. Knopf, 2003.

Sterling, Dorothy. *The Outer Lands,* revised ed. New York: W. W. Norton & Company, 1978.

Svenson, Henry K. and Robert W. Pyle. *The Flora of Cape Cod.* Brewster, MA: The Cape Cod Museum of Natural History, 1979.

Tiner Jr. and Ralph W. *A Field Guide to Coastal Wetland Plants of the Northeastern United States.* Amherst: The University of Massachusetts Press, 1987.

Whatley, Michael E. *Common Trailside Plants of Cape Cod National Seashore.* Eastham, MA: Eastern National, 1988.

APPENDIX C:
INFORMATION SOURCES

GOVERNMENT AGENCIES

Cape Cod National Seashore
Headquarters
(508) 349-3785

Salt Pond visitor center
(508) 255-3421

Province Lands visitor center (seasonal)
(508) 487-1256
www.nps.gov/caco

Cape Cod Regional Transit Authority
(800) 352-7155;

"The Breeze" buses and shuttles
(508) 790-2613
www.thebreeze.info

Cape Cod towns
Barnstable
(508) 862-4000
www.town.barnstable.ma.us

Bourne
(508) 759-0600
www.townofbourne.com

Brewster
(508) 759-0613
www.town.brewster.ma.us

Chatham
(508) 945-5100
www.town.chatham.ma.us

Dennis
(508) 394-8400
www.town.dennis.ma.us

Eastham
(508) 240-5900
www.eastham-ma.gov/home

Falmouth
(508) 548-7611
www.town.falmouth.ma.us

Harwich
(508) 430-7513
harwichma.virtualtownhall.net/home

Mashpee
(508) 539-1400
www.ci.mashpee.ma.us/pages/index

Orleans
(508) 240-3700
www.town.orleans.ma.us

Provincetown
(508) 487-9560
www.provincetowngov.org

Sandwich
(508) 888-0340
www.sandwichmass.org

Truro
(508) 349-7004
www.truro-ma.gov

Wellfleet
(508) 349-0300
www.wellfleetma.org/home

Yarmouth
(508) 398-2231
www.yarmouth.ma.us

Manuel F. Corellus State Forest
(Edgartown and West Tisbury,
   Martha's Vineyard)
(508) 693-2540
www.mass.gov/dcr/parks/southeast/
   corr.htm

Martha's Vineyard Transit Authority
(508) 693-9440
www.vineyardtransit.com

Martha's Vineyard Land Bank Commission
(508) 627-7141
www.mvlandbank.com

Massachusetts Division of Fisheries and Wildlife
(hunting information)
www.mass.gov/dfwele/dfw

APPENDIX C: INFORMATION SOURCES

GOVERNMENT AGENCIES (continued)

Monomoy Island National Wildlife Refuge (Chatham)
(508) 945-0594
www.fws.gov/northeast/monomoy

Nantucket Islands Land Bank
(508) 228-7240
www.nantucketlandbank.org

Nantucket Regional Transit Authority
"The Shuttle"
(508) 228-7025
www.shuttlenantucket.com

Nickerson State Park (Brewster)
(508) 896-3491
www.mass.gov/dcr/parks/southeast/nick.htm

South Cape Beach State Park (Mashpee)
(508) 457-0495
www.mass.gov/dcr/parks/southeast/socp.htm

The Steamship Authority
(boat to Martha's Vineyard and Nantucket) Vehicle reservations
(508) 477-8600, (508) 693-9130

Fast Ferry reservations (no cars)
(508) 495-3278
www.steamshipauthority.com/ssa

OTHER ORGANIZATIONS

Appalachian Mountain Club, Southeastern Massachusetts Chapter
www.amcsem.org

Ashumet Holly Wildlife Sanctuary (Mass Audubon), Falmouth
(phone contact through Long Pasture Wildlife Sanctuary, Barnstable)
(508) 362-1426
www.massaudubon.org/nature_connection/sanctuaries/ashumet_holly/index.php

Bay State Cruise Company
(Boston–Provincetown ferry)
(866) 903-3779, (508) 487-9284
www.provincetownfastferry.com

Boston Harbor Cruises
(ferry service between Boston and Provincetown)
(877) 733-9425, (617) 227-4320
www.bostonharborcruises.com/ptown_main.html

Cape Air (flights to the Cape and Islands from Boston, New Bedford, and Providence)
(800) 352-0714, (508) 771-6944
www.flycapeair.com

Cape Cod Bird Club
(phone contact through Cape Cod Museum of Natural History)
(508) 896-3867
www.massbird.org/ccbc

Cape Cod Chamber of Commerce
(508) 362-3225
www.capecodchamber.org

Cape Cod Museum of Natural History
(508) 896-3867
www.ccmnh.org

Cape Cod Outdoors (camping info)
www.capecodoutdoors.com

Cape Cod Pathways
(Barnstable County)
(508) 362-3828
www.capecodcommission.org/pathways

Cape Cod Recreation (camping info)
(508) 430-0185
www.capecodrec.com

Cape Cod Web
www.capecodweb.com

Capt. John Boat Lines (ferry service between Plymouth and Provincetown)
(508) 747-2400
www.provincetownferry.com

Continental Express
(flights to Nantucket from Newark)
(800) 523-3273
www.continental.com

APPENDIX C:
INFORMATION SOURCES

OTHER ORGANIZATIONS *(continued)*

Falmouth–Edgartown Ferry
(ferry service between Falmouth and Martha's Vineyard)
(508) 548-9400

Felix Neck Wildlife Sanctuary (Mass Audubon), Edgartown, Martha's Vineyard
(508) 627-4850
www.massaudubon.org/nature_connection/
sanctuaries/felix_neck/index.php

Freedom Cruise Line *(ferry service between Harwichport and Nantucket)*
(508) 432-8999
www.nantucketislandferry.com

Friends of the Cape Cod National Seashore
(508) 349-3785, x402
www.fccns.org

Green Briar Nature Center
(Sandwich)
(508) 888-6870
www.thorntonburgess.org/Green%20
Briar.htm

Historical Society of Old Yarmouth
www.hsoy.org

Hy-Line Cruises
(ferry service from Hyannis to Martha's Vineyard and Nantucket)
(800) 492-8082, (508) 778-0404
www.hy-linecruises.com

Insider's Guide: Cape Cod, Nantucket & Martha's Vineyard
www.insiders.com/capecod

Island Airlines *(flights to Nantucket from Hyannis)*
(800) 248-7779, (508) 228-7575
www.islandair.net

Island Queen *(ferry service between Falmouth and Martha's Vineyard)*
(508) 548-4800
www.islandqueen.com

Long Point Wildlife Refuge, West Tisbury, Martha's Vineyard
(508) 693-3678
www.thetrustees.org/pages/
315_long_point_wildlife_refuge.cfm

Lowell Holly Reservation, Mashpee and Sandwich
(508) 679-2115
www.thetrustees.org/pages/
316_lowell_holly.cfm

Martha's Vineyard Chamber of Commerce
(800) 505-4815, (508) 693-0085
www.mvy.com

Mashpee Wampanoag Tribe
(508) 477-0208
www.mashpeewampanoagtribe.com

Massachusetts List of Endangered, Threatened, and Special Concern Species
www.mass.gov/dfwele/dfw/nhesp/
nhrare.htm

Menemsha Hills Reservation, Chilmark, Martha's Vineyard
(508) 693-3678
www.thetrustees.org/pages/
322_menemsha_hills.cfm

Nantucket Airlines
(flights to Nantucket from Hyannis)
(800) 635-8787, (508) 228-6234
www.nantucketairlines.com

Nantucket Chamber of Commerce
(508) 228-1700
www.nantucketchamber.org

Nantucket Conservation Foundation
(508) 228-2884
www.nantucketconservation.com

Outermost Adventures
(boat shuttle to North Monomoy Island and South Beach, Chatham)
(508) 945-5858
www.outermostharbor.com

APPENDIX C:
INFORMATION SOURCES

OTHER ORGANIZATIONS (continued)

Patriot Party Boats (ferry service between Falmouth and Martha's Vineyard)
(800) 734-0088, (508) 548-2626
www.patriotpartyboats.com

Peter Pan–Bonanza Bus Lines
(bus service to Cape Cod from many East Coast cities)
(888) 751-8800
www.bonanzabus.com

Plymouth and Brockton (bus service to Cape Cod from Boston and Logan Airport)
(508) 746-0378
www.p-b.com

Rip Ryder (boat shuttle to North Monomoy Island and South Beach, Chatham)
(508) 945-5450
www.monomoyislandferry.com

Sheriff's Meadow Foundation
(Martha's Vineyard)
(508) 693-5207
www.sheriffsmeadow.org

Smart Guide (car-free-travel planner published by the Cape Cod Chamber of Commerce)
(888) 332-2732
www.smartguide.org

The 300 Committee (Falmouth)
(508) 540-0876
www.300committee.org

US Airways Express (flights to the Cape and Islands from many East Coast cities)
(800) 428-4322
www.usairways.com

Wampanoag Tribe of Gay Head
(Aquinnah)
(508) 645-9265
www.wampanoagtribe.net/pages/index

Waquoit Bay National Estuarine Research Reserve
(508) 457-0495
www.waquoitbayreserve.org

Wasque Reservation, Chappaquiddick Island, Edgartown, Martha's Vineyard
(508) 627-7689
www.thetrustees.org/pages/372_wasque.cfm

Wellfleet Bay Wildlife Sanctuary (Mass Audubon), Wellfleet
(508) 349-2615
www.massaudubon.org/nature_connection/sanctuaries/wellfleet/index.php

Woods Hole Research Center
(508) 540-9900
www.whrc.org

INDEX

INDEX

INDEX

INDEX

INDEX